Praise for
Heal Your Child from the Inside Out

"*Robin is on the cutting-edge of a movement. Heal Your Child from the Inside Out will help you understand why our children are suffering from more food sensitivities and chronic health issues than ever, and Robin will teach you how to care for children in a way that supports their individual personality and physiology so they can be vibrantly healthy and happy. I'll be purchasing this book for every parent I know! Robin's teachings have benefited all three of my children beyond measure, and I know they will do the same for your family.*"

— **Erin Day Cox**, wellness expert and author of *One Hot Mama: The Guide to Getting Your Mind and Body Back After Baby*

"*Robin Ray Green has written an essential handbook for the practice of holistic pediatrics, conceptually rooted in the profoundly illuminating paradigm of Traditional Chinese Medicine. She has creatively expanded upon the model of Five-Phase (Element) types first articulated in Between Heaven and Earth to produce an inspiring and eminently practical guide for parents and providers who seek to foster the optimal growth, health, and happiness of their children and patients. Kudos for a job well done!*"

— **Efrem Korngold, OMD, L.Ac.**, co-author of *Between Heaven and Earth: A Guide to Chinese Medicine*

"*Robin Ray Green has given parents a comprehensive guide to raising their children using the time-tested framework of Chinese medicine's Five-Phase model. As a pediatrician working with children for the past 30 years, I have found this approach highly effective in helping parents understand the unique characteristics and needs of their children. Robin's book complements the work that Efrem Korngold and I have developed over the years and makes it her own. Her humor and compassion come across in every page as she teaches how to recognize a child's Dominant Element and manage imbalances and health challenges. She offers practical solutions that include massage, diet, acupressure, and mindfulness practices that will heal your child from the inside out, which is a welcome resource for any parent.*"

— **Stephen Cowan, M.D., FAAP**, author of *Fire Child, Water Child: How Understanding the Five Types of ADHD Can Help You Improve Your Child's Self-Esteem and Attention*

"With _Heal Your Child from the Inside Out,_ Robin Ray Green has produced a new and trailblazing type of book that takes Five-Element theory and makes it accessible and applicable for modern parents. This book gives parents practical strategies to implement a personalized holistic health regimen for their children, empowering them to improve health through focused alterations in the core components of healthy child development: diet, lifestyle, and emotional regulation. Robin also helps parents see how to best understand, communicate, guide, and direct their children based on their constitutional types and subsequent natural tendencies. Further, she provides insight and techniques for integrating that so-often neglected area of nurturing: healthy touch. This book provides a practical approach for integrating the best of ancient and modern theories for child rearing, and I have no doubt that parents who incorporate the ideas presented will see improvements in the health and well-being of their children and their families as a whole."

— **David W. Miller, M.D., FAAP, L.Ac., Dipl OM.,** founder of East-West Integrated Medicine, LLC

"Ever wonder why so many kids these days seem to have so many chronic health issues? Why are so many children falling into an 'unwellness gap,' where they aren't majorly sick but aren't completely well? Robin draws on her experience as a pediatric acupuncturist and a mother to explore why this is happening to our kids, and what can be done about it. _Heal Your Child From the Inside Out_ will teach you a 'new' way to look at your child, based on the 'old' teachings of Traditional Chinese Medicine. With Robin's fun yet practical approach, you will understand your children's unique nature, how best to nurture them, and how to create a custom healing plan to optimize their wellness. This is a must-have guide for parents to understand the unique nature of each child and how to best support them in order to be happy, healthy, and well. Robin is on a mission to improve children's health. This book will help parents do just that."

— **Elisa H. Song, M.D.,** holistic pediatrician and founder of Whole Family Wellness

"With her brilliant mastery of the Chinese Five-Element System, as well as her compassionate understanding from her own experiences as a parent, Robin Ray Green is the perfect guide to show you how to read your child's individual map. This book is a wonderfully practical and comprehensive 'user's manual' for your child's optimal health!"

— **Jean Haner,** author of *The Wisdom of Your Child's Face: Discover Your Child's True Nature with Chinese Face Reading*

heal your child
from the
inside out

Hay House Titles of Related Interest

YOU CAN HEAL YOUR LIFE, the movie,
starring Louise Hay & Friends
(available as an online streaming video)
www.hayhouse.com/louise-movie

THE SHIFT, the movie,
starring Dr. Wayne W. Dyer
(available as an online streaming video)
www.hayhouse.com/the-shift-movie

Awakened by Autism: Embracing Autism, Self, and Hope for a New World,
by Andrea Libutti, M.D.

Ignite the Light: Empowering Children and Adults to Be Their Absolute Best,
by Vicki Savini

10-Minute Recipes: Fast Food, Clean Ingredients, Natural Health,
by Liana Werner-Gray

*Veggie Mama: A Fun, Wholesome Guide to Feeding Your Kids Tasty
Plant-Based Meals*, by Doreen Virtue and Jenny Ross

*The Wisdom of Your Child's Face: Discover Your Child's True Nature with
Chinese Face Reading*, by Jean Haner

All of the above are available at your local bookstore,
or may be ordered by visiting:

Hay House USA: www.hayhouse.com®
Hay House Australia: www.hayhouse.com.au
Hay House UK: www.hayhouse.co.uk
Hay House India: www.hayhouse.co.in

heal your child
from the
inside out

The 5-Element Way to Nurturing Healthy, Happy Kids

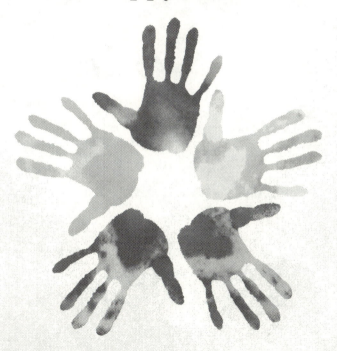

Robin Ray Green, L.Ac., MTCM

HAY
HOUSE

HAY HOUSE, INC.
Carlsbad, California • New York City
London • Sydney • New Delhi

Published in the United States by: Hay House, Inc.: www.hayhouse.com® • *Published in Australia by:* Hay House Australia Pty. Ltd.: www.hayhouse.com. au • *Published in the United Kingdom by:* Hay House UK, Ltd.: www.hayhouse. co.uk • *Published in India by:* Hay House Publishers India: www.hayhouse.co.in

Project editor: Nicolette Salamanca Young • *Interior design:* Bryn Starr Best
Cover design: Karla Baker, karla.baker@mac.com • *Interior photos:* Kendra Knight, kendraknightphotography.com • *Interior illustrations:* Rashid A. Rehman • *Chart 7.1:* Illustration on pg. 181 courtesy of earseeds.com

Library of Congress Cataloging-in-Publication Data

Names: Green, Robin Ray, date, author.
Title: Heal your child from the inside out : the 5-element way to nurturing
   healthy, happy kids / Robin Ray Green.
Description: Carlsbad : Hay House, Inc., 2016.
Identifiers: LCCN 2016023576 | ISBN 9781401948696 (paperback)
Subjects: LCSH: Parenting. | Child rearing. | BISAC: HEALTH & FITNESS /
   Acupressure & Acupuncture (see also MEDICAL / Acupuncture). | FAMILY &
   RELATIONSHIPS / Parenting / General.
Classification: LCC HQ755.8 .G727 2016 | DDC 649/.1--dc23 LC record available at
https://lccn.loc.gov/2016023576

ISBN: 978-1-4019- 4869-6

1st edition, October 2016

Printed in the United States of America

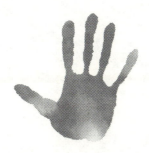

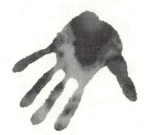

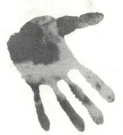

*This book is dedicated
to my boys, Noah and Nate.
Thank you for inspiring me
to be a better mom and a better
healer, and to help other kids just
like you around the world.*

CONTENTS

YOUR 5-ELEMENT WAY
COMMUNITY

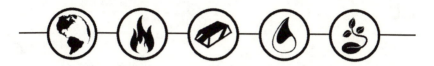

It's amazing what can happen when you embark on a journey to heal your child from the inside out. There will be many changes, challenges, and breakthroughs. When I started on my journey, it was a bit lonely. There was so much to learn, and I had to figure it all out through trial and error.

Now you don't have to make this journey alone! You'll find a community with tips, information, and healing inspiration at www.robinraygreen.com. I offer numerous free resources to help you blend Eastern and Western medicine in your everyday life, including:

- **Free articles and videos** on how to treat common childhood conditions naturally.
- **The free companion kit to this book**, which includes the questionnaires, quizzes, healing program template, and the *Chinese Wellness Massage Video*.
- **Instructional photos** to teach you how to do acupressure and tuina massage at home.
- **Online classes and guides**, with step-by-step directions for using Traditional Chinese Medicine to heal your child.
- **A community of passionate and supportive parents** who offer encouragement and guidance. Their numerous stories of how their children have healed are what keep me inspired!
- **My newsletter**, which will keep you in the loop on my latest blog posts, webinars, free events, live classes, acupressure guides, and more.

Visit www.robinraygreen.com today.

FOREWORD

Robin and I had an instant connection from our first conversation. She had applied to join my first mastermind group in which I mentor women and help them reach more people by growing their online presence, speaking, and writing books. I immediately knew we would connect on both a professional and personal level, but I had no idea of the powerful impact Robin was going to have on my life.

Robin had been healing children at her clinic with acupuncture and Traditional Chinese Medicine (TCM). She wanted to broaden her reach and teach other TCM practitioners and acupuncturists her unique and powerful way of working with children. However, I recognized that her work with children was profound and needed to be shared with the masses! My mission was to help Robin also teach parents how to help their own children heal through diet, acupressure, massage, and the tenets of TCM.

I know that moms out there are desperate for what Robin has to teach because I am the mom of three young children myself. I hear what other moms struggle with and worry about. We regularly discuss why so many of our children suffer from eczema, food sensitivities, and allergies when we feel like we feed our kids mostly healthy food. We notice that none of us or our friends experienced these health issues as children, yet they seem commonplace today. We wonder: What the heck is going on?

As moms, we want to do what's best for our children, and thankfully Robin is on a mission to help all parents understand the truth. She is on the cutting edge of a movement that I hope and pray will lead to higher-quality food choices for all people. As parents, we have to educate ourselves so we know how to feed our families; we must stop supporting food corporations' profits at the expense of our children's health. There is simply too much at risk. With approximately 17 percent of our children being obese and more kids than ever suffering from food sensitivities, allergies, diabetes, depression, and other maladies, we need to change our culture around food and wellness.

As time went on and I really started working closely with Robin and understanding her business, I clearly saw her absolute passion for her work, her sincere love of children, and her intuitive healing gifts. I knew I had to have my middle child, Elena, see her in person.

A few years prior to meeting Robin, Elena had broken her leg badly when she fell off playground equipment as a two-year-old. After a surgery to set her broken bones, she received a rigorous round of antibiotics and painkillers, and had been struggling with serious stomach issues and constipation ever since. The constipation and resulting discomfort, moodiness, frustration, and suffering she experienced when she wouldn't go to the bathroom for weeks at a time became intolerable. Our well-meaning pediatrician told me to avoid constipating foods. He said we'd probably struggle for years, and we would just have to continue giving her laxatives.

I felt like a failure as a mother. Elena was constantly in anguish, and I was helpless. It was heartbreaking to witness, and it was negatively impacting the lives of our entire family. Our doctor's recommendation just did not feel right to me, but I thought I had tried everything. I was frustrated and miserable because it seemed as though there was nothing I could do to make things better for my child.

After the six-hour drive to Robin's clinic, Elena and I were greeted with warmth. Robin's immediate connection with my daughter was beautiful. She established an instant level of trust and ease as she conducted a thorough exam of both me and Elena. (In fact, I recognize many of the questions we were asked in the incredibly useful quizzes in this book.)

Robin helped me understand the root of Elena's issues. She explained that the strong dose of antibiotics and trauma of the accident had nearly wiped out Elena's healthy gut flora. Together, we developed a treatment plan that felt feasible, including massage, diet modifications, and probiotics. Although we were eating pretty healthy and mostly organic foods, Robin showed me where we could do better. We've slowly changed our entire family's diet, and it has been a hugely positive and beneficial experience for everyone. There are always more ways that we can improve, but we do the best we can and improve little by little every day. As a single mother raising three kids while working more than full-time, I truly believe it is possible for *any* family to implement Robin's teachings.

I am beyond grateful for the healing Robin was able to help me facilitate in Elena's health. She went from a moody, grumpy, pale little girl with dark circles under her eyes to a bright-eyed, energetic, rosy-cheeked, and truly delightful child who is absolutely thriving in kindergarten. The diet and lifestyle changes felt like an effort in the beginning, but seeing such a profound transformation in my child has made me a lifelong believer.

Working with Robin in person is a transcendent experience; reading *Heal Your Child from the Inside Out* is a close re-creation of that magic. I love that Robin considers the whole child and doesn't just treat the symptoms. It simply makes sense. I read this book intently, taking notes and enjoying the process. This invaluable book is a download of her genuine brilliance, magic, and expertise that is sure to help families all over the world. It is a book that I will be referencing constantly and sharing with all my parent-friends. The more we know, the better we can protect our families and offer every child what they need to be vibrant, happy, and successful in their own unique ways.

I now have a fuller understanding of many of the topics Robin discussed with me during our appointment. I've also gained a better appreciation for who each of my children are and how I can best care for them based on their Dominant and Influential Elements. It was amazing to see the traits and descriptions of each of my children's personalities described so accurately. I now recognize that it's just the way they are wired and part of their innate physiology. With the wisdom of the Five Elements, I can feed and care for each of my children in a way that gives them the greatest opportunity for optimal wellness.

I am excited for you to learn more about your child, and possibly even yourself. I love all children, and nothing makes me more excited than imagining the positive transformation that your child could make as a result of reading this book. Good luck, and lots of love to you and your family in your journey to vibrant, thriving, full wellness!

— With love,

Erin Day Cox, wellness expert and author of
*One Hot Mama: The Guide to Getting Your
Mind and Body Back After Baby*

INTRODUCTION

I never imagined that I'd become a pediatric acupuncture specialist. When I earned my master's degree in Traditional Chinese Medicine (TCM), my holistic training focused on treating adults with acupuncture and herbs. My journey to this specialty started simply from a desire to help my infant son heal from a severe case of eczema that wasn't responding to Western medical treatments. Only after I began treating him with acupuncture, herbal medicine, and dietary changes did his eczema begin to resolve.

As I shared my son's story with my patients, they'd tell me that their children suffered from conditions that I knew could be treated with holistic care and acupuncture. Inspired by my child's recovery, my patients began to bring their kids in for treatment, too. And as word spread about how I had helped these kids with conditions such as colic, constipation, cough, and ear infections, I began seeing even more children in my office—and this is how my family practice was born. The lives of thousands of kids around the world have been dramatically impacted by my own practice as well as by the acupuncturists whom I trained to work with kids.

But I never would have arrived at this place of helping kids heal naturally if my son's poor health hadn't served as a wake-up call. It went something like this . . .

"He'll probably grow out of it . . . eventually," the pediatrician said dismissively. I had been hoping for answers, or at the very least effective treatment, for the angry red rash that had been spreading over my 18-month-old son's body nearly his entire life. Was "Do nothing" really all his pediatrician had to say? Despite visits to specialists and full medical evaluations, we were no closer to figuring out what was causing Noah's eczema and even further from curing it. I imagined Noah suffering his entire life with an awful rash all over his body. I wondered about all the things he might miss out on and feared his school years would be torturous. *He'll grow out of it eventually?* Waiting wasn't an option!

I found myself wondering how we had gotten to that point. The pediatrician's dismissive answer stirred up deep fears about Noah's future—and doubts about every decision my husband and I had made as parents! As first-time parents, we were afraid of making the wrong decisions about Noah's health, and we trusted our pediatrician because we felt he knew best. He had gone through medical school, had thousands of hours of training in pediatrics, and had treated hundreds of children before Noah. We wanted to be "good" parents, so we went along with all of our pediatrician's recommendations. There were times when I was uneasy about the medical choices we made, but I had been raised not to question the doctor. I followed the program, even though my instincts were screaming at me to make a different choice.

I'm not saying that our pediatrician was a bad doctor. On the contrary, he did the best he could for us within the medical framework he was trained in. However, his treatment plan was incomplete because: (1) it didn't treat the root cause of Noah's eczema, (2) it was a one-size-fits-all treatment and didn't account for Noah's unique nature or the other issues he was having, and (3) it didn't address him as a whole child; it just addressed the illness. If we are to achieve deeper healing and promote the overall well-being of our children, we need an approach that addresses not only the illness but also the *whole child* who has the illness.

Please don't misunderstand what I'm saying here. It's not that Western medicine is bad or should be abandoned. Rather, it's quite the opposite. Drugs and medical procedures can intervene and rescue a child from a life-threatening situation. We should take full advantage of the solutions modern medicine has to offer. But we should also remember that drugs and procedures are incredibly potent. They can help, but they can also harm and may have long-term negative consequences. It's important to use Western medicine wisely, when needed, along with other approaches.

The Traditional Chinese Medicine Approach to Healing and the Unwellness Gap

There's a saying that rings true for me and many parents: "You're only as happy as your least-happy child." In the beginning, my husband and I were so worried about Noah that we fell into the same mode of thinking as the doctor; our singular focus became monitoring Noah's eczema. We were unhappy, worried, and afraid. We needed answers to restore balance and harmony to Noah's health as well as our entire family.

Suddenly, a lightbulb went on. I realized that due to my fears, I had neglected the TCM perspective of viewing illness within the context of the whole person. I had the training and the knowledge base; it was up to me to wade through the overwhelming amount of information on diet, herbs, and other natural remedies. We didn't have to wait anxiously for Noah to outgrow his eczema; we could take charge and solve the mystery of his worsening condition. Our pediatrician had done the best he could with the Western medicine tools he had, but now it was time to venture into the world of natural healing.

First, I reminded myself that, for the most part, Western medicine views illness as an entity separate and distinct from the person, something to be identified and eliminated with drugs or medical procedures. TCM takes a patient-centered approach, viewing illness in the context of the whole person—body, mind, and spirit—and coming up with a treatment plan that addresses the symptoms along with the underlying cause of the imbalance.

It's not surprising that the one-size-fits-all approach of Western medicine falls short for many kids. When I started on this journey, I had no idea that millions of other children were unnecessarily suffering with conditions like Noah. I now call this state the "unwellness gap": when a child is not totally sick and needing to be hospitalized, but not totally well, either. These children suffer from inflammatory conditions and chronic low-grade illnesses that warrant repeated trips to the doctor, yet there's no pill that can cure them.

In the United States, the number of children falling into the unwellness gap has been on the rise, especially in the past 25 years.[1,2,3] Approximately seven million children suffer from asthma, contributing to missed school days and hospital visits.[4] More than six million children suffer from food allergies, the numbers increasing 50 percent between 1997 and 2011.[5] Food, digestive, skin, and respiratory allergies increasingly affect children and interfere with their ability to lead normal lives in which they can run, swim, and play. All combined, the number of children who suffer from asthma, allergies, autism, and ADHD comes to more than 20 million![6] That's one in three American kids affected by these chronic conditions. This doesn't even include all the children suffering from frequent acute illness—those who are sick more often than well with ear infections, upper respiratory infections, chronic runny noses, and coughs.

I find these numbers shocking, and sadly, this is just the tip of the iceberg. For every child who is diagnosed, there are many more who suffer silently. Medicine has advanced so much in the past century, but despite greater access to well-baby care, vaccines, and increased spending on health care, our children are getting sicker. If you're a parent, you intuitively know this. How many of your friends have kids who are frequently ill or who have asthma, food allergies, eczema, autism, or ADHD? Compare that with the number of kids who had the same conditions when you were growing up. It's frightening, right?

Noah's illness was my wake-up call to start asking deeper questions. Why have we been able to virtually eradicate many infectious diseases like polio, diphtheria, smallpox, chickenpox, and mumps, while the rates of contemporary chronic illnesses are skyrocketing? I thought chronic illness was due to a lifetime of unhealthy eating, lack of exercise, or exposure to environmental pollution and toxins. So why do so many babies and young children suffer from them when their bodies are brand-new?

In my quest to answer these questions and understand Noah's eczema, I went down the rabbit hole. I researched every possible cause I could think of and discovered fascinating connections to genetics, environmental toxins, pollution, and pesticides. I learned how dramatically our food supply has changed in the last few decades, and the ways that this affects gut flora, immune function, and ultimately our health.

It was eye-opening to realize what is happening to our environment and diet. It seems that the way we've treated planet Earth—polluting our air, water, soil, and food—is having a devastating effect on our health, especially our kids' health. For a while, I was in denial and wanted to pretend I didn't know these things, but you can't "unknow" what you know.

Even though it was scary to realize how many things could have contributed to Noah's having an inflammatory skin condition at a mere three months of age, I realized it wasn't my fault. If your child is suffering from a chronic illness, *it's not your fault!* When it comes to chronic illness, there often isn't one identifiable cause, but many possible causes. Some of them we can control, like our diet and the chemicals that we bring into our home. Others we have no way of controlling, like the hidden toxins we're exposed to and the pollution in our air and water.

Because children increasingly suffer from contemporary chronic childhood illnesses that were virtually unheard of 40 or 50 years ago, we can't always rely on the wisdom of our parents to help us manage these issues. When you are the first generation in a family to face these conditions, where can you turn for help in overcoming these challenges? Fortunately, the ancient wisdom of TCM can help us understand where we've lost our way. It can help us bring balance and harmony to the lives of our children and our entire family.

While there are various schools of thought within the TCM tradition, I was drawn to the Five-Element system, which is an ancient paradigm for understanding how a person's temperament, physical health, emotional health, and spiritual health are all interrelated. I felt it was the most comprehensive way to understand who my child is, his distinct personality and body type, and the imbalances causing his eczema. The Five-Element system allowed me to take a more holistic perspective of Noah's illness and formulate a plan to treat the whole, amazing, beautiful baby that was Noah.

How This Book Will Help You

As a licensed acupuncturist, which is the most common type of TCM practitioner in the United States, I've been on the front lines helping hundreds of children in my clinic. I personally know the grief and guilt parents experience when their child is suffering and they don't know what to do. *Heal Your Child from the Inside Out* is about empowering you, as the parent, to create your own treatment plan and find a health-care team that addresses not only your child's illness, but your child as a whole person—body, mind, and spirit.

If you're reading this book, you're probably the type of parent who doesn't want to sit around waiting for your child to "outgrow" illness, either. You want to find answers that will help you solve your child's problem now. You don't want to address just the symptoms; you want to heal the underlying cause. You love your child more than anything in the world, and you want to do your best for him. Trying something new, different, or unconventional can be a little bit scary if you don't feel supported. Using outside-the-box solutions is likely to stir up fears about being judged negatively by your doctor, friends, or family members. These feelings can be magnified if your partner doesn't support your desire to try natural remedies. You may fear the struggle of making changes to your child's diet or lifestyle and making him seem different from other children.

I totally get it, because I was in the same position. What you'll find in this book are practical, commonsense solutions any parent can implement. Even though TCM is relatively new in the Western Hemisphere, it is based on thousands of years of empirical observation with a solid framework for diagnosing and treating illness. The tools you'll gain will help augment whatever Western medical treatments your child is already undergoing. You can have the best of both worlds!

In this book, I'll start by introducing you to the basics of Traditional Chinese Medicine and the Five Elements. Then I'll help you identify your child's Dominant Element and provide you with proactive strategies for nurturing this element to bring out the best in your child—physically, emotionally, and spiritually.

Once you discover your child's Dominant Element, we will dive into Five-Element diagnosis. When there are imbalances in any one of the Five Elements, specific health problems will arise. I'll help you recognize when these imbalances occur and provide strategies for prevention and guidelines for healing.

Finally, I'll outline specific strategies that you can implement *immediately* to support your child's body and facilitate healing. The focus will be on diet, lifestyle, massage, and how best to nurture your unique child to better health.

With the Five-Element way of thinking, you'll learn how to connect with your child where he is and honor his unique individuality so you can create a harmonious family life. You'll also learn how to navigate the issues in our modern lifestyle and environment that can affect your child's health.

Healing your child is not just a journey for the child; it's a journey of rediscovery for the entire family. When your child is happy and well, all those worries, fears, and doubts dissolve. Instead of focusing on your child's illness, you can bring back love, trust, and fun to your entire family. Are you ready to get started?

CHAPTER ONE

How the Five Elements Influence Your Child

Each child comes into this world with a distinct nature, unique as a snowflake or fingerprint. Parents with more than one child know how true this is. Even as newborn babies, your children are inherently different. Their preferences and needs are as individual as they are—and their medicine should be, too!

Traditional Chinese Medicine (TCM) takes a patient-centered approach to healing and is one of the oldest known theories of body-mind-spirit medicine. It is a system of healing that has been developed and refined over the past 4,000 years through observing the patterns found in nature to explain how the body, mind, and spirit are interrelated and constitute our health. In the United States, there are many different schools of Oriental medicine with varying emphases on specific traditions. My framework for TCM and the Five Elements is based on the training I received in my master's program, my clinical practice, and my journey to heal my own family. In this chapter, I distill the most important aspects of TCM to give you a basic understanding of how to use this medicine, but what I share only scratches the surface of this ancient knowledge.

Qi and Meridians and Our Health

One way we understand how every process of the body-mind-spirit is interrelated is through the TCM concept of qi and meridians. The word *qi* (pronounced "chee") can be translated in many different ways, but its most common definition is: a vital force or energy that permeates the heavens above and the earth below. I like to think of it as a universal building block with many manifestations, depending on what it is connected to: the universe, nature, the physical body, the mind, or the spirit. Qi is the thing that connects human beings to the universe at large. There are many different forms of qi in the human body that serve different purposes.

In the body, qi flows within specific pathways called meridians. There are 12 main meridians distributed around the body internally and externally. They branch off into smaller and smaller channels, carrying qi to every organ, tissue, and cell in the body. It's similar to the way arteries distribute blood to the whole body, but in the case of meridians, they carry qi.

Just as the nervous system or the circulatory system comprises a vast network that covers and connects the entire body, so does the meridian system. The difference between the meridian system and other body systems is that it connects the physical body to the mind and spirit as well.

The way our qi connects to our body, mind, and spirit is a complex relationship that involves many different manifestations of qi that connect and support one another. To put it simply, each main meridian connects to an organ, and that organ's manifestation of qi relates to what we think of as the mind or spirit. For example, the heart is connected with the mind.

Another important concept in TCM is that our health is a manifestation of flow. In order to be healthy and stay alive, our breath must flow in and out, our blood must flow in our arteries and veins, and nerve impulses must flow from synapse to synapse. In the same way, our qi must flow unimpeded in our meridians. If our qi becomes congested in one area due to trauma, whether emotional or physical, it can affect the body, mind, and/or spirit, thereby leading to pain, illness, or depression. Qi can also become congested or stagnant due to poor diet, lack of sleep, stress, or any number of issues that build up over a long period.

Think of it this way: a blockage in the flow of qi is like a kink in a hose. If the water in the hose can no longer reach the flowers, the plants will wilt and eventually die. To save them, we must understand what's causing the kink, and then we can unkink the hose and restore the flow of water to the flowers. In this way, restoring the flow of qi in the meridians creates balance in the body, which can resolve illness and restore well-being.

The Whole Child According to TCM

In order to treat the whole child, we must see the child as a triad of body-mind-spirit because, according to TCM, your child's health is the result of the interactions among all three. The health and vitality of a child cannot be gauged merely by the status of her physical body. The terms *body*, *mind*, and *spirit* are often glibly used and glossed over, but to me they have a very deep meaning, especially in terms of healing. When I use these terms in the context of the whole child, it signifies the three aspects of healing that must be balanced for a child to thrive.

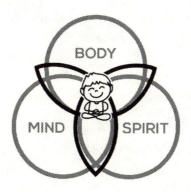

Figure 1.1: The Whole Child

In order to closely examine the intricate relationships linking the body, mind, and spirit, we will begin with a seemingly healthy child. This child's body may be healthy by modern standards, but if she has anxiety about going to school or difficulty getting along with other kids, or if she feels unsafe in any environment, this will eventually lead to physical and/or emotional issues. For example, she may suffer from chronic stomachaches, but doctors may not be able to find a definitive cause even after extensive medical testing. The stomachaches are real and debilitating, but they're more than a simple physical problem that can be healed with drugs. In cases like this, the mind and spirit connection is not being addressed. Doctors have done what they can to address the body, leaving the parents on their own to explore other avenues to help their child find relief.

A Western doctor will perform a physical exam and inquire about the nature, location, and associated symptoms to rule out the more serious causes of stomachache that would require medical intervention—an important first step in addressing the condition. However, to understand the entire story of the illness from the whole-child perspective, we need to go deeper. We'll look at the body-mind-spirit aspects of this problem and ask a different set of questions to find out what's happening in the child's life that could be causing the illness. We'll assess her mood, energy, sleep, lifestyle, relationships, and any other precipitating factors to give us additional clues as to what is going on. At the same time, we need to acknowledge that the symptoms are very real and not dismiss them as "all in her head."

From a holistic perspective, the most obvious physical cause of a stomachache would be the child's diet. What has she been eating lately? Could her symptoms be due to a change in her diet or a new sensitivity to a food she once tolerated? This would be an obvious first question for a medical doctor, too, but once the results of a standard IgE food allergy test are found to be negative, food is often dismissed as a cause of pain. However, a negative IgE test is not the end of the story. The IgE immune response is not the only way the immune system can react to a food, and many children experience abdominal pain related to foods they're sensitive to.

In addition, a child's mental and emotional state will affect her physical health. Is she struggling with a particular subject at school? Is she having problems with a teacher or other students? Could the stomachaches be from anxiety? Are her parents getting a divorce? Has she recently lost a loved one or pet? As we begin to explore new aspects of the same problem, it can help us resolve the stomachaches in a way that honors the child's experience and makes her stronger in the long run.

Can you see now how we address the whole child by using body-mind-spirit medicine? Bringing balance to restore optimal health is the ultimate goal of the whole-child approach in TCM. Now, let's take a look at how exactly we address each aspect of the whole child: body, mind, and spirit.

The Body

The body is the aspect that is most familiar to us. It represents the child's physical health. In TCM, we assess the health of the body by reviewing the function and interplay of many factors, including:

- Immune function
- Digestive function
- Energy level
- Sleep quality and quantity
- Appetite and thirst
- Physical activity
- Physical developmental milestones

When the body is healthy, the immune system is strong and the child is not prone to frequent illness or repeated infections. When the child does get sick, which is a normal part of developing a healthy immune system, the illness resolves in a timely manner. The child has regular, daily bowel movements that are well formed and easy to expel. Food is easily digested, and there are no signs of nausea, gas, bloating, or stomachaches. The child has the right amount of energy, neither too much nor too little. The child falls asleep easily and, upon waking, feels energized and ready for the day ahead.

The quality and quantity of food eaten are extremely important for creating robust physical health in our children. Nutrient requirements vary significantly, depending on the age of the child. Regardless, food should be organic, with as little processing as possible. Care should be taken to avoid artificial colors, flavors, and preservatives because they're toxic to the brain and body. Meals should be eaten at regular intervals to ensure stable blood sugar levels. The child's appetite should match activity level and caloric requirements, not causing her to eat too much or too little. When balanced, the child won't have any excessive cravings for sweets, dairy, salt, or carbohydrates, nor will she be an extremely picky eater, either.

When a TCM practitioner evaluates a child's health, she will ask about the symptoms of illness and pose general health-assessment questions that address various aspects of body, mind, and spirit. This allows her to determine the pattern of imbalance that is impacting the child's overall health.

The Mind

The mind represents the child's thinking, emotions, and mental clarity. Of course, you should expect different levels of mental clarity and emotions depending on your child's age. For instance, it is normal for a three-year-old to throw the occasional tantrum, whereas the same behavior would be concerning in a ten-year-old.

Depending on the age of the child, the following aspects of the mind are assessed in TCM:

- Mental clarity
- Attention and focus
- Memory, learning, and cognition
- Feelings and fluidity of emotional states
- Interpretation of environmental stimuli through the five senses
- Intellectual developmental milestones
- Mental habits and thought patterns
- Outlook or perception of events

As children get older, emotions, mental habits, and perception of events become incredibly important to the child's overall health and happiness. Even at a young age, children can begin to worry and have obsessive thoughts. Over time, these become mental habits that can lead to clinical anxiety and depression.[1]

It's normal for everyone's emotions to vary throughout the day or week, but we need to be able to move through emotions, positive or negative, so we don't get stuck and suffer the ill effects physically. (Remember the importance of flow!) Stagnant emotions can lead to physical symptoms and contribute to illness. Staying in a state of anger or frustration for long periods of time, for instance, can raise blood pressure and contribute to other symptoms in the body, like headaches. Asthma is a wonderful example of how emotions, good or bad, can trigger physical symptoms. It is well documented that anger, anxiety, and even laughter can trigger an asthma attack.[2,3]

When a child's mind is healthy and strong, he can think clearly and move through emotions easily. He develops positive mental habits that allow resilience under stress. He'll be less likely to develop mental illness later in life. Attention and focus are balanced, making it easy for the child to learn and remember new ideas. He can make good decisions and learn from his mistakes. He is flexible as life events unfold and maintains a positive outlook even in the face of challenges.

The Spirit

In TCM, spirit is defined as "the force that animates and perpetuates living beings and organisms."[4] It is believed that a person's spirit is reflected in his vitality and can be seen when he is thriving. Physically, we can "see" the manifestation of spirit by looking at the vibrancy in the eyes; like the English proverb, it is believed in TCM that the eyes are truly the windows of the soul.

In TCM, the body is the vessel of the spirit. As TCM expert and author Giovanni Maciocia explains, "If the spirit is strong, the person has a clear voice that projects outward well, the eyes and complexion have lustre, the expression is lively, the mind is clear and alert, the person walks with an erect posture and has a naturally optimistic, enthusiastic and mentally strong attitude."[5]

Spirit is difficult to capture in words because, to me, it's a feeling or knowingness that comes from the energy exuded by the child—that inherent state of wonder, presence in the moment, and unconditional love for all things.

In my TCM practice, I assess my patients' spirit by listening to them in terms of the following:

- Happiness and optimism
- Creativity and playfulness
- Resilience and ability to overcome adversity
- Life purpose and meaning
- Ability to share one's unique gifts with the world
- Feeling of connection to Spirit
- Empathy and compassion

When a child's spirit is strong and healthy, she can dream big dreams. She's happy and optimistic about life, which gives her resilience in the face of adversity. She goes through her day with a sense of wonder at what she experiences. She is present in the moment. She feels connected to Spirit—to something greater than herself—which gives her life meaning and purpose and inspires love, empathy, and compassion for others.

One thing's for sure: we can clearly see when a child's spirit is broken. The eyes lack luster, and these kids don't dare to hope or dream. Their drawings are filled with darkness, reflecting a world of sadness and instability. Their broken spirit can be seen and felt as emanating from deep within their core. They can't see that they matter or that life has any meaning.

Unfortunately, the world is full of influences that don't support us in nurturing our spirits. As spiritual teacher Marianne Williamson writes, "We're not raised in a society that asks, 'What are your gifts, and how can they make the world a more beautiful place?' We're usually asked something more like this: 'What will you do to make a living?' This knocks us out of our natural rhythm, because the soul simply doesn't think that way."[6]

Nurturing our children's spirit is very important for their lifelong health and must be taken into account when we're searching for the root cause of any illness.

To Treat the Disease, Find the Root

There's an old Chinese saying: "To treat the disease, find the root." In other words, while we need to treat the symptoms of an illness, for true healing we must also address what's causing the symptoms at the root. The beauty of TCM is that it gives us a framework for understanding patterns that contribute to and create disease. It can help us find the path back to better health.

One way TCM explains the pattern of an illness is through what is called "root and manifestation" theory. It sounds complicated, but it's really quite simple. Envision an oak tree. The tree shows us a balanced way to live our lives. It takes care of itself. It consumes the minerals it needs from the earth, takes in water, and transforms the light and warmth of the sun into the right amount of energy to create as many branches, leaves, and acorns as it needs. The tree is a model of balance.

Below the surface of the earth, invisible to the eye, are the roots of the tree. Aboveground are the trunk and branches, which can be thought of as the manifestation of the roots. The quality and health of the branches are the manifestation of the quality and health of the roots.

If a tree is suffering an illness, you can sometimes cut off the affected branches and the problem is solved. But if the illness is coming from the roots, you're not really solving the problem by cutting off the branches; the tree is still sick.

In straightforward cases, treating the symptoms of an illness (cutting off the branches) makes complete sense. Let's go back to our example of the child with a stomachache. If the pain is due to an *H. pylori* bacterial infection, then giving oral antibiotics will fix the problem. But if this child is having stomachaches and no bacterial infection can be found, further investigation is necessary to identify the root. A doctor might prescribe an antibiotic to see if it would help, but that would be like cutting off a branch when the problem is really with the root. Furthermore, when you focus on just cutting off branches (treating symptoms), the weakened state of the tree can create other problems.

As an illness progresses, especially a case of chronic illness, the root and manifestation can become numerous and complicated. Determining the root cause (or causes) is key to unraveling the pattern of symptoms. Then a comprehensive treatment plan can be developed to address both the underlying cause of an illness and its symptoms.

The Five Elements

The Five Elements in TCM intertwine and balance one another to keep our tree (our body) healthy from root to branch. The Five-Element system is a diagnostic tool that, along with root and manifestation theory, can help us understand the interacting forces that shape our physical, mental, emotional, and spiritual health. To understand the Five Elements, we must first look at where they originated and what each element comprises. Then we can examine how an understanding of your child's Dominant and Influential Elements can help you heal him as a whole child.

The Five-Element system theory originated with early Chinese philosophers around 476 to 222 B.C. They were students of the laws of nature, and they keenly connected with and observed their environment to deepen their understanding of the rhythms and interrelationships of nature. Their goal was to help mankind attune to the natural order of things, to understand the rhythms of the earth and live in harmony with it. They saw that each element has its own unique "medicine" that it gives freely to support the natural order of life. Early Chinese physicians used the patterns they observed in nature to describe physiological processes in the human body and understand what was happening in the body when the elements were out of balance and creating disease. They also used these patterns to better understand our emotions, mental state, and relationship to the world around us.

The Five Elements are Wood, Fire, Earth, Metal, and Water. Just as we sometimes use metaphors from the outer, physical world to describe what goes on in our inner world, we can use the earth's ecosystems to understand the personal ecosystem within our body-mind-spirit triad. Just as in nature, our personal ecosystem contains all Five Elements that must remain in balance for us to be happy and healthy.

Let's look at how the Five Elements must be balanced for any type of ecosystem to flourish. Envision a beautiful forest. There are mountains made of rock that contain ore (Metal). There are a clear lake and a stream (Water), and bountiful trees and shrubs (Wood) grow in rich soil (Earth). The sun (Fire) is the spark that gives life to all things.

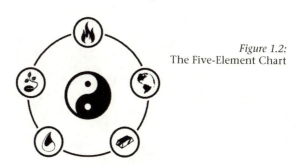

Figure 1.2:
The Five-Element Chart

When all Five Elements in the ecosystem are balanced, the forest flourishes, providing a habitat with plentiful food and water where all creatures thrive. The trees grow strong and tall, providing food and shelter for animals and wood for fires. Fire, in the form of the sun, provides the necessary energy for all things to grow. Fire burns wood, generating ash to nourish the earth, which creates rich, fertile soil in which plants can grow. The earth contains ore that can be refined by humans into metal and shaped into useful objects for survival such as bowls, axes, knives, and spears. Metal provides trace minerals that enrich water and help sustain plants and animals. Rain nourishes the plants and soil and furnishes water that flows through the land, providing a habitat for fish and water for the birds and other animals.

If any one of the Five Elements becomes imbalanced, it will affect the entire ecosystem. Let's say lightning strikes and starts a forest fire. The trees provide ample fuel for Fire, which can easily blaze out of control. Without Water to stop the Fire, it will easily consume the entire forest, displacing the creatures in the ecosystem, ruining the habitat, and creating a wasteland. Whereas if it were to rain sufficiently, Water would put out the Fire and the ecosystem would easily be able to recover. In their natural order, the elements keep one another in check. Each element has a role to play to keep the ecosystem balanced.

In the personal ecosystem in our bodies, each element must be balanced in the same way. Each element has unique, inherent qualities that it shares within our personal ecosystem to make sure that we stay balanced and healthy. In our personal ecosystem, each element is associated with a particular temperament, mental state, emotion, physical archetype, season, color, smell, taste, and sound, to name just a few.

Each ecosystem on the planet has an element that dominates it. For instance, Wood dominates forest ecosystems and Water dominates marine ecosystems. The Dominant Element shapes the landscape and makes the ecosystem unique. In the same way, our personal ecosystems are dominated by one element that influences how we grow and develop into the unique individuals we are. This Dominant Element shapes our personality, our temperament, and how we interpret the world around us. It becomes the lens through which we view the world and determines how we're likely to act within it.

In TCM, we use the Five Elements by breaking down the traits of each element into a system of correspondences that we can utilize to understand ourselves better, promote health, and resolve illness. While the Five Elements have been used to treat adults for centuries, the idea of using it to understand and aid the normal growth and development of our children is a more modern notion, put forth by pediatric acupuncture experts Efrem Korngold, OMD, L.Ac.; Stephen Cowan, MD; and Harriet Beinfield, L.Ac. (Their seminal works in the field can be found in the Recommended Resources at the end of this book. If you're interested in understanding your own Five-Element type, I highly recommended reading *Between Heaven and Earth: A Guide to Chinese Medicine* by Beinfield and Korngold.)

While my predecessors' groundbreaking work on Five-Phase typing inspired my continued study and helped inform my understanding of how each type manifests, *Heal Your Child from the Inside Out* is the culmination of my own study, observations, and use of the Five Elements with my own children and the children I work with in my clinic. What I present here is how I have personally come to interpret and use the Five Elements.

With the Five Elements as our framework, we can truly address our children as the beautiful, whole people that they really are: body, mind, and spirit. Once we recognize how our world is shaped through the framework of the Five Elements, we find that its application goes beyond health and healing to all areas of life. It can give us concrete strategies for making changes that positively impact our children. It can also help us meet our children's unique needs and understand how the needs of each child are different. It allows us to figure out how to parent each child in a way that honors her unique nature and brings harmony to the family. It helps us teach our children how to deal with adversity so they can become resilient. The Five Elements also help us understand our own nature as individuals and as parents, thereby recognizing when our child's needs differ greatly from our own.

Your Child's Dominant and Influential Elements

Each child comes into this world with a unique combination of the Five Elements. One element will predominantly shape your child's nature and the way he responds to his environment. This is his Dominant Element. By knowing a child's Dominant Element, you can understand his strengths and weaknesses, predict the types of illnesses he is prone to, and determine which season he'll need the most support to keep him healthy.

In my own experience, ignoring Noah's Dominant Element was what contributed to his being chronically ill, because we were always treating the symptoms instead of addressing the underlying cause. Conversely, identifying Noah's Dominant Element has allowed me to systemically heal him and our entire family.

Below is a chart that shows some of the elemental correspondences and the traits that might be demonstrated in a child who has each Dominant Element:

	Wood	Fire	Earth	Metal	Water
Prone to	Headaches, muscle spasms, behavior problems	Anxiety, sleep issues, overdoing it	Digestive problems, overeating	Asthma, colds, skin issues	Low-back pain, body aches, bedwetting
Gifts	Curiosity, drive	Creativity, charisma	Caring, helping others	Vision, ability to see big picture and little details	Imagination, innovation, creativity
Challenge	Anger, irritability, managing emotions	Focus, impulse control, moodiness	Obsession, worry, people-pleasing	Flexibility	Structure, punctuality, fitting in
Emotional Tendencies	Anger	Joy	Worry	Grief	Fear

Table 1.1: General Characteristics of Each Element

In some children, the Dominant Element is evident early on and is consistent as the child gets older. These children are pretty easy to spot since they embody the nature of their element in everything they do. They are the easily recognizable archetypes: the Wood child who is the team captain, the Fire child who is the star of the drama club, the Earth child who is Mommy's little helper, the Metal child who wins the spelling bee, the Water child who's a natural artist.

Because children are still growing and developing, their Dominant Element may not be obvious, and they may present a blend of two or three archetypes. They may seem to resonate with one element at certain times and then resonate with another in different situations. I believe this happens because, in addition to the child's Dominant Element, there may be one or two other elements significantly influencing how the Dominant Element is expressed. I call these the Influential Elements.

Influential Elements soften or bolster certain traits of the Dominant Element, changing how it is expressed. This is what makes each Fire child different, each Water child different, and so on. As you read through the descriptions of each element, you'll begin to see which element is your child's Dominant Element and which others might be Influential Elements.

The Wood Child—Explorer, Pioneer, Adventurer

The energy of Wood is one of growth, movement, and expansion. From the moment the seedling sprouts, it's in a constant state of action, always expanding and pushing its boundaries. You can try to fence in a forest, but it's hard to contain. Wood will find a way. If not kept in check by firm boundaries, Wood will easily take over. When in balance, Wood can pioneer new frontiers. The Wood child is very energetic, curious, and adventurous, representing the nature of Wood in the ecosystem.

James is the perfect example of the Wood child. His mother says, "From the moment he could crawl, it seemed like James was always on the go. It wasn't too long after crawling that he figured out how to climb the stairs and get out of his crib. We quickly realized we couldn't take our eyes off him, because he was always getting into something." James's mom is a Metal type, which is more quiet and reserved, so she found it exhausting trying to keep up with him.

Early in life, you'll often hear the Wood child saying, "Me do it." He loves to discover how things work on his own. When he sets his mind on something, he will find a way to get it—like climbing on a chair to reach the cookie jar on the counter. Wood babies and toddlers are superactive, wiggly, and always on the move. Their curiosity drives them to explore their environment and get into things they shouldn't. They are the early crawlers, the explorers, the "Don't restrain me in this car seat or I'll scream" kind of babies. Child locks and other childproof devices are simply challenges for them to overcome.

As the Wood child gets older, he will continue to be extremely active. His well-developed motor coordination may make him a natural athlete. Because of his competitive nature, he'll be attracted to team sports and driven to win. A natural leader, he'll often become a team captain and have other kids looking up to him. No matter what, he needs physical outlets in order to manage his energy and feelings, which will enable him to stay balanced.

Curiosity and a drive to figure things out often lead to early entrepreneurial endeavors. The Wood child might start his own business at a young age, whether it's a lemonade stand or a lawn-mowing service—he is highly motivated. But curiosity can also lead to constant questioning of parents and teachers. He likes to challenge himself and push boundaries to see how firm they are with authority figures.

When faced with an obstacle he can't overcome, the Wood child often responds with frustration and anger. His moods may be more volatile and intense than those of children with other Dominant Elements. He is used to things coming easily to him and can find it especially difficult when he can't understand something, lashing out at those closest to him. Because of his persistent nature, he can also get frustrated when he doesn't get his way and may argue about even the smallest thing until his parents relent. Providing positive discipline and firm boundaries can help keep the Wood child from ruling the roost.

When the Wood child is not in balance, he can look wild and out-of-control. His parents may have difficulty disciplining him, and he may be defiant. In extreme cases, he may lash out physically. At school, he may have trouble staying in his seat, following the rules, and taking his turn. Wood children, when out of balance, are more likely to be diagnosed with attention-deficit/hyperactivity disorder (ADHD) with predominant hyperactivity or Oppositional Defiance Disorder (ODD).

The physical archetype of the Wood child is tall and lean or short and compact, but always muscular. His face tends to be narrow and long and may be described as rectangular-shaped, often with a prominent jawline and protruding brow.[7]

David needs to be constantly in motion and is a quintessential Wood child. His mom and dad say that while he's an intense kid, he is a joy to parent because he's pretty fearless and throws himself wholeheartedly into everything he does. He loves intensely, he competes intensely, and he even sleeps intensely. His mom says, "Early on, we realized he needed firm yet loving boundaries to keep him safe and to help us keep him in check." Because he has strong opinions, his parents have allowed him to ask them why they have made a decision he disagrees with, and while he may present a counterargument, he's not allowed to continue arguing or back talk once a decision is final.

The Fire Child—Free Spirit, Entertainer, Performer

The energy of Fire is magnetic, stimulating, and transformative. In the ecosystem, Fire is represented by the sun, which draws all living things to it. The warmth of Fire has a transformative quality; its light and heat is the catalyst for life-giving photosynthesis for plants. A fire burns wood, turning it into ash that nourishes the Earth's soil. The light and shadows of a fire dance and play, but fire still needs to be contained so it doesn't blaze out of control and quickly burn itself out. Therefore, on the more active side of the continuum, the Fire child is bright and vibrant and seeks lots of stimulation. The magnetic quality of these kids comes from their Fire energy. Even as babies and toddlers, they exude a spark that attracts others to them.

Steve describes his daughter Sophia, a Fire child, as strong-willed and determined—a force of nature. "She's a very personable, likeable kid who thrives in social situations. She craves stimulation and engagement and has a yearning to learn." As with many Fire children, Steve finds that Sophia has an insatiable appetite for creative growth and is always ready to go from one project to the next. She is always making things and doing crafts, but it can be challenging to find activities that will hold her attention for very long because she quickly masters the basics and is ready for more. Steve says that "sometimes boundaries are difficult to maintain as Sophia tends to push boundaries because of her need for growth."

As a baby, the Fire child equally loves to be held and to explore her environment, seeking the stimulation of new objects. When she finds something that grabs her attention, it may hold her captive for quite some time, as she tends to get wrapped up completely in everything she sees and feels. Once bored, she will be ready to explore again, seeking new things to focus on. She is delighted to play games like peekaboo and give you a beautiful smile and delightful giggle. She enjoys the stimulation of new sights and sounds.

As the Fire child gets older, she still wants her parents to entertain her and play with her, which can sometimes be exhausting for them. She's a very active and engaging kid who likes constant movement and is easily distracted by bright, shiny objects. When you take her to the store, she may want to touch and explore things, her curiosity pushing the boundaries. Her parents may be constantly telling her, "Look with your eyes, not your hands." But she can't help herself; her curiosity and sensation-seeking behaviors can make it hard not to touch things.

She experiences life through her senses more fully than other children because she is more open and receptive. She likes to explore how things feel, sound, smell, and taste. Because she experiences life through her senses so strongly, her reactions to things may be stronger and more intense than those of other children. Her mood may shift rapidly from laughing and giggling to crying and being upset and then back to laughing again. Distraction is a great way to move her attention away from something that's upsetting her.

A Fire child may enjoy entertaining you. She may show an interest in dance, art, singing, and acting as a way to channel her creative spirit. She recharges by being around people and loves being surrounded by friends and family. She can't wait to share every detail of her day at school as soon as she sees you! Her need for constant activity needs to be balanced with quiet time so she doesn't get overstimulated.

When faced with obstacles, the Fire child may easily lose her temper in the heat of the moment. She may have an explosive temper when things don't go her way. She may also tend to become anxious and fearful when facing a difficult or new situation. Because she craves excitement and creativity, she can easily become bored and act out.

When the Fire child is out of balance, she'll act like a class clown or a drama queen. When out of balance, her demanding nature may manifest in "spoiled brat" behaviors; she may pout or refuse to talk to you when she doesn't get her way. The smallest slight may seem like the end of the world to her. Because she's easily distracted, she may have difficulty staying focused or following simple instructions. She may be prone to anxiety and overthinking, which can make it difficult for her to fall asleep. At school, she may be impulsive and overly talkative and may have difficulty focusing on the task at hand. She may complain that school is boring. The Fire child is more likely to be diagnosed as having ADHD with impulsivity.

The physical archetype of the Fire child has well-developed shoulder muscles and small, elegant hands and feet. You'll often observe a sparkle in her eyes; her complexion has a healthy pink flush. A Fire child may often have dimples and a pointed chin. Curly hair is very common as well.[8]

Rose is a beautiful Fire child with cute dimples and long, curly red hair. She loves to perform, and going to circus camp was the highlight of her summer. In fact, she loved it so much that her parents bought her a unicycle so she could practice performing at home. Rose enjoys being the center of attention. She loves being recorded on video and watching herself over and over again. A bright and charismatic child, she makes friends wherever she goes. Her mom says, "Rose has brought so much joy into our home. She can be a firecracker and challenging at times, but she also brings fun into the most mundane chores. It's all about channeling her energy!"

The Earth Child—Helper, Peacekeeper, Mother

The Earth is the center of life. The Earth is a grounding force, openly giving whatever is needed to keep harmony and balance in the ecosystem, asking only for what it needs to survive in return. Silent and steady beneath us, the Earth is always supporting, giving, and helping living things. The Earth is there when you need it, yet almost invisible in the background. In the middle of the Five-Element continuum, the Earth child is a natural helper and caregiver, as represented by the energy of the Earth. He is friendly, outgoing, and talkative but doesn't necessarily enjoy being in the spotlight.

You can always recognize Earth babies because they are the cutest, chubbiest, most lovable infants. They have plump cheeks that you just can't resist squeezing, and robust, thick builds. People are drawn to the warm nature of Earth babies and toddlers, and they are adored by everyone. Earth babies love being attached to their primary caregiver at the hip. For example, if their primary caregiver is their mom, they may cry or fuss when handed over to Dad or Grandma, although they'll smile and play with them as long as they're in Mom's arms. As toddlers, Earth children are more likely to cry for Mom when dropped off at preschool.

My son Nate is an Earth child. When he was a baby, friends and family used to call him Chubbers because of his sweet cheeks. In the grocery store, he would smile and wave to people who would inevitably come over to coo at him and tell me how cute he was. As he got older and I went back to work, he had a really hard time. He would follow my car down the street, and we'd wave at each other and blow kisses until finally I had to turn the corner. Even today, he is an affectionate and loving child who is extremely attached to his family, including our dog, Ginger.

As the Earth child gets older, he is Mommy's helper and enjoys assisting with chores and caring for other children. At a young age, he may feel responsible for others and take his duty to care for plants or animals very seriously. He loves to eat and explore new foods and enjoys activities like cooking and baking. Family gatherings are a favorite time for the Earth child. Even at an early age, he shows compassion for other living things and may cry and get upset when a beloved pet bug dies. He usually likes to play with stuffed animals, and as he gets older, he may hound you for a pet of his own.

A natural peacekeeper, the Earth child wants to make sure everyone is getting along well. He is very loving and affectionate and will be attached to whoever cares for him. He has lots of friends and is very talkative. Some might describe him as a chatterbox. He may love to sing and hum at home but is reluctant to be the center of attention. Despite his many friends, transitions each school year may be a little tough because he'll be attached to his teacher and reluctant to move on.

While your Earth child may go with the flow, he can also get worried about his family, friends, and pets and is reluctant to be away from them for very long. When faced with a challenge, the Earth child will need time to think things over. While he likes to mentally sort through problems to figure out all the possible solutions, this can also lead to worry and obsessive thoughts. It's important to check in with him to help him sort through his thoughts and emotions and bring his attention back to the present moment.

When the Earth child is out of balance, he will be prone to worry and to have obsessive thoughts. Because of his need to get along well with others, he may not voice his own needs and may easily be taken advantage of by others. This can lead to low self-confidence, which may be perceived as neediness. At school, the Earth child can easily become overwhelmed by tasks that require him to sort a lot of data, and when out of balance he may become disorganized and messy.

The physical archetype of the Earth child is a larger, thicker, and stockier body. His face is wider and rounder, and his head may be larger.[9]

Joy is Mother's little helper and is always there with a thoughtful word or hug. She writes inspirational messages on Mom's whiteboard and is always at the ready to cheer people up or to help someone in need. When I did a house call to treat her brother after he had an emergency appendectomy, Joy was at his side the entire time. She'd been so worried about her brother that she got a stomachache and stayed home from school to be with him.

At the young age of nine, Joy headed up the planning of her mom's surprise birthday party. She even contacted all her mom's friends to invite them to the event. It is important to Joy that everyone in the family get along. Her favorite times are family gatherings for special occasions, when she can walk around being the hostess, making sure everyone is settled and happy. She enjoys looking after her younger cousin, doting on her as if imagining what it will be like to have her own kids one day. Joy is very outgoing and talkative when she's comfortable, but she can also be shy and quiet until she's feeling comfortable in a situation.

Metal—Wizard, Visionary, Father

Metal is probably the most difficult element to place in our ecosystem. Traditional Chinese philosophers use mountains to represent the strength and visionary qualities of Metal. However, while Metal originates as ore in the earth, in that state it lacks a useful form. When heated, it becomes malleable and can be molded into any shape. When cooled, its rigid shape becomes its rightful purpose. At its essence, Metal creates order from disorder.

I like to envision Metal as a beautiful silver bowl that continues its purpose of creating order from disorder. It can hold water or items to create organization. Being Metal, the bowl is very sensitive to the environment. If left in the sun, it absorbs the heat. If dipped in a cool river, it not only holds water but also absorbs the cold. It is a receptacle for everything around it—a sensitive indicator of what is going on in the world.

The Metal child is also like an open receptacle. She will easily reflect your emotional state back to you. She is sensitive to her environment and feels things, including the energy of others, very deeply. It is by receiving all this information that she becomes a natural visionary, able to see all the little details but also the big picture.

My son Noah is a classic Metal child. For the most part, he was an extremely easy baby, though it seemed as if, from the day he was born, his sensitivity dial was set to 10! When he was an infant, if a fire truck drove by our house with sirens blaring during his nap time, that was it. Noah would be awake and inconsolable, and we'd have to start his nap routine all over again. Now, at age 12, he is a very well-behaved and articulate young man. He loves solving puzzles and figuring out patterns, and his favorite activity is using Legos to create his own unique inventions.

As a baby, the Metal child is very easygoing and thrives on routine and ritual. She is a caring, loving baby and is very attached to her parents. The Metal baby may be easily disturbed by loud noises, such as loud vehicles passing your house. Sudden changes in schedule may throw a Metal child out of balance. She may have a hard time if she misses a nap or goes too long without eating. Metal children are generally calm and very well-behaved, wanting nothing more than to please their parents and do as they're told. It only takes being told once or twice not to touch something, and she will leave it alone. Door locks on your kitchen cabinets may not even be necessary because she already knows the rules.

As a Metal child gets older, she's active, but not as active as Fire and Wood children, who keep their parents on the go all the time. Instead, she enjoys a balance of activity and quiet time. She seeks to understand the order of the world. Routines help her understand what's coming next, so she can prepare herself for the flow of the day or week. Although easygoing, even at a young age she may be particular about many things, especially foods, and sensitive to textures and tastes. Metal children explore the world through all their senses, so new environments can be overwhelming for them; they need extra love and support from their parents as they adjust. The Metal child is likely to have a small group of close friends. She is loving, funny, and outgoing with close relatives and friends, but shy with strangers until she gets to know them.

When faced with an obstacle, the Metal child seeks to find a pattern so she can solve the problem. Her parents may need to explain how things work in detail, and on a very adult level, so she can gain a clearer understanding. She can get frustrated to the point of tears when she can't figure things out. The Metal child has a strong sense of righteousness. She sees the need for rules and has a strong sense of responsibility. In fact, she can take too much responsibility for things, and this can weigh on her and lead to obsessive thinking and negative thoughts. If she gets fixated on things beyond her control, she may feel down. It's important to make sure that she doesn't take things too seriously and can be flexible in her thoughts and problem-solving skills.

When out of balance, the Metal child becomes rigid and inflexible. At school, this can manifest as perfectionist tendencies that make her a slow worker who easily falls behind and becomes overwhelmed as the class switches from activity to activity. She may obsess over rules that have been broken or fixate on something she's not allowed to have. She can become stubborn, and her strong-willed nature can easily outlast your resolve. Parents should be careful before making threats, because she may push you to follow through on what you've said.

The physical archetype of the Metal child is a thin and narrow body with a small head and square jaw. The Metal child may tend toward a pale complexion and a larger nose.[10]

Matty is the sweetest, most well-behaved little boy. He is very cooperative, and once he knows the rules, you rarely have to tell him what to do. The rhythm of his day keeps him in the flow, and knowing what is coming next helps him feel secure. If you forget the order of his day or leave something out of his routine, he's sure to remember and let you know. He sees all the little details and has a fantastic memory. Legos, puzzles, and train tracks are his favorite toys, and he loves to put things together in order to figure

out how they work. You can see him puzzling things out and creating the big picture from the little pieces. He is very discerning
and particular about things. Matty's parents say, "He was an easy
baby, and he's been easy to parent so far. But we have to be flexible
in our decisions because forcing him to do something he doesn't
want to do can be a disaster."

Water—Creator, Innovator, Dreamer

The energy of Water is that of flow; it easily bends and moves
with the sway of the land. Water can be still and reflective on the
surface, but concealed underneath is a rich inner world where fish,
algae, rocks, and other entities share a complex coexistence. Water
is quiet and serene, yet given the right conditions, it can become
a force of nature, drastically changing the landscape in ways we
never could have imagined. At the end of the Five-Element continuum farthest from the Wood child, the Water child goes with
the flow, but he also has a very creative mind and is likely a deep
thinker with a rich inner world.

Allison's daughter, Noelle, is a Water child who came into the
world with a whole different energy and presence that were apparent from the very beginning. "We sensed her old soul in her big,
beautiful eyes," Allison says. "Her quietness was apparent early
on and most notable in contrast to her older sister, a Wood child.
She was easy from the beginning, and she was able to find a way
to self-soothe so she didn't need a lot of comforting." Allison adds
that even when Noelle is in the room, she doesn't take up the
kind of space that her Wood sister does. She doesn't overdrama-
tize situations but instead internalizes what she's experiencing.
However, because of her quiet nature, she easily gets lost in the
shuffle. At the farmers' market, she can wander off and disappear
in the crowd, lost in her own world. When Noelle began going to

preschool, she tended to sit in the corner and watch the others. She was easily overwhelmed and would often cry. Sometimes it can be difficult for her to switch from one activity to another. And her fear of the dark and loud noises can make it hard for her to go to sleep. Overall, Noelle has a wisdom beyond her years and a very different perspective on life.

As a baby, the Water child is the most easygoing. She is content to lie or sit on the floor taking in all that she sees. She is a master observer, although when motivated, she will begin to explore her world as all the other elements do. She is very loving and attached to her parents. She's shy and may not want to talk to or make eye contact with people she doesn't know.

As the Water child gets older, she feels more deeply than other children, often understanding emotional nuances in profound ways. Parents may describe their Water child as an "old soul." She can occupy herself for hours in her own creative world, exploring her deeper thoughts and feelings. She will likely have a few close friends and be content with staying home. A little bit of social activity is all she needs to feel connected with others. Too much affection, talking, and stimulation can overwhelm her. Parents need to give her space to be alone.

The Water child tends to have a timid nature and may be scared to try new things or activities that are very stimulating. Quick movements, noisy fireworks, or jumping too high on a trampoline can easily overwhelm her senses. Raising your voice will intimidate her, and fear often makes her withdraw and hide. She may do the same when faced with challenge or upset. When her thoughts and feelings are too much for her to handle, she needs time to be alone to work things out in her own mind. It can be frustrating for parents when she hides in the closet or under blankets instead of talking things through.

The Water child moves to the beat of her own drum. Constructs of time may be difficult for her to follow, as she can't sense the passage of time the way other people can. She may be difficult to hurry along, so make sure to budget plenty of time for her to get ready for school or errands. The structure and pace of school may also be difficult; she tends to get so caught up in what she's doing that she often doesn't realize the class has already moved on to the next activity. Because she's quiet and doesn't make a fuss, her teacher may not realize that she's behind in her studies, and she may need one-on-one help to get through her lessons.

When out of balance, the Water child is off in her own world. She has difficulty being on time and doing well in structured activities. Because she doesn't mind being alone, she may have trouble making friends and building relationships. She may feel that she doesn't "fit in" with other kids and can become a loner at school. Lacking motivation, she may fall behind in her studies and is more likely to be diagnosed with ADHD with predominant inattention. She may become bored and daydream in class and miss vital information about her assignments or forget to turn in her work even though she has completed it.

The physical archetype of the Water child is a compact, round, somewhat stocky body with a round face, broad cheeks, and a darker complexion.[11]

Grant is perfectly content staying home after school and playing with his Legos. He can spend hours getting lost in his own imaginary world or reading a book. The worst thing in the world for Grant is running errands or being in structured after-school activities; he'd much rather be at home. While he likes riding his bike and playing soccer, he is most balanced when he has alone time after school.

Unlike his Earth sister, Grant needs to know why he has to do something or how he'll benefit. While generally easygoing, he can also be stubborn if he's not on board with an activity. Grant has no problems being on time or working within a structured environment; however, trying to force him to do things quickly usually has the opposite desired result.

Determine Your Child's Dominant Element

Determining your child's Dominant Element involves two main steps. In step 1, you take the Yin/Yang Qualities Quiz to determine whether he is more yin or more yang. Since children often show characteristics of multiple elements, this will help you start narrowing it down so you can find where your child falls on the Five-Element continuum. In step 2, you'll take the Five-Element Questionnaire. Be sure to read my tips to get the most accurate results.

When determining your child's Dominant Element, the most important thing is to look at the characteristics that are strongly manifesting at this moment in time. As a child grows up, it's possible that the Dominant and Influential Elements will swap places due to a variety of environmental and lifestyle factors. You can best help your child by understanding and supporting his *current* Dominant Element.

Step 1: Determine Your Child's Yin/Yang Nature

Yin and yang theory is a way to organize and plot the Five Elements on a continuum, thereby allowing you to quickly begin to narrow down the elements that most resonate with your child's way of being in the world. This will then help you determine your child's Dominant and Influential Elements.

Figure 1.3: Yin/Yang Symbol

You may be familiar with the yin/yang symbol as shown here. In Traditional Chinese philosophy, yin and yang represent two fundamental energies or forces that are present in the universe.

Although yin and yang theory is more complex than what I'll present here, you can think of yin and yang as opposite yet complementary forces. On one side, yang represents energies that are light, bright, hot, active, expanding, strong, clear, upward, and outward. On the other side, yin represents the opposite: energies that are dark, dim, cold, still, contracting, weak, turbid, inward, and downward.

Yin and yang are not absolutes, but relative opposites that are defined by the perspective of the observer. For example, we know what dark is only in the context of its opposite: light. How dark a room seems is determined by the observer's point of view. Think of going from a brightly lit room into a dark one. When you enter the dark room, it appears dim and you can't make anything out. But a person already in the dark room may be able to see fairly well, and the night-light in the room may seem bright to her.

We can use these complementary yin and yang forces to categorize the Five Elements on a continuum.

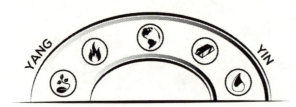

Figure 1.4: The Five-Element Continuum

As you can see, the elements are arranged from left to right, from most yang to most yin. On the left (yang) side are Wood and Fire, and on the right (yin) side are Metal and Water. In the middle is Earth, which has both yin and yang qualities, sometimes in almost equal quantities. This can make the Earth child very difficult to type.

Children falling on the yang side of the continuum will have more of the yang characteristics, such as super-high energy and activity. Children on the yin side will have more of the yin characteristics, such as being more easygoing and having a slightly lower activity level (although all kids are active). In addition, notice how the color of the borders of the continuum gradually grows darker as you move from left to right. This represents the idea that there isn't a distinct demarcation separating each element. Instead, the elements gradually transition from one to the next.

To determine your child's yin or yang nature, take the quiz below. Please be aware that your perspective influences what you consider to be yin and yang. For example, when examining the type of energy your child may have, the observation is informed by your own Dominant Element. To a Water parent, which is most yin on the continuum, an Earth child may seem really yang. But when you compare an Earth child with a Wood child, who is truly superactive, constantly on the go and unable to sit still, you see that she's really not all that yang.

Yin/Yang Qualities Quiz

Read the descriptors below and circle the qualities that best describe your child in comparison with other children. Does your child tend to be more yin or yang with regard to the characteristics below?

Yin	Yang
Quiet	Loud
Reserved	Outgoing
Often feels cold	Often feels hot
Active, but enjoys quiet	Superactive
Easygoing	Demanding
Introverted	Extroverted

If you circled more characteristics in the first column, your child has more yin qualities, so he may be an Earth, Metal, or Water child. If you circled mainly characteristics in the second column, your child has more yang qualities, so he may be a Wood, Fire or Earth child. If he has equal amounts of yin and yang qualities, he may be an Earth child or have a combination of yin and yang Dominant and Influential Elements.

Step 2: Determine Your Child's Dominant Element

The second step is to take the Five-Element Questionnaire in Appendix A. When taking the quiz, be sure to keep these five tips in mind to help you get the most accurate results.

1. Consider how your child acts in different settings.

As you check off the characteristics that resonate with your child's way of being in the world, think about how your child acts across multiple settings, including school, social gatherings, sporting events, and home.

2. Remember that your child is a unique combination of all Five Elements.

Remember, each child is a manifestation of all Five Elements, so he will at times resonate with different characteristics. Don't be surprised if you're checking off a few traits under each element.

3. Know that your child may resonate with two elements very strongly.

You may also find that your child resonates very strongly with two elements. It may even be difficult for you to determine which one is your child's Dominant Element. If this happens, it means your child has both a Dominant Element and an Influential Element. In this case, observe your child in different settings to see if you notice patterns of behavior. In addition, read through the descriptions of the elements that best describe your child in Chapters 1 and 2. All these steps should give you some clarity about which element is Dominant and which is Influential. Remember, there's no right or wrong here. It's simply a matter of seeing which element best represents the way your child is in the world.

4. Keep your child's age in mind.

While the questionnaire is geared to children of all ages, it's important to keep in mind your child's age when answering questions about certain behaviors. Ask yourself if what you're seeing is age appropriate as compared with other children of the same age and developmental stage. For instance, a tantrum that would be concerning for a child of 10 would be developmentally appropriate for a child at age three. Once your child begins elementary school, it will be easier to determine his Dominant Element.

5. *Know that the Dominant Element is reflected in three key areas.*

If you have any difficulty determining your child's Dominant Element, in addition to the steps above, you'll want to closely observe three key areas of behavior that most accurately reflect your child's Dominant Element. They are:

- Activity level: How active is your child in comparison with other children?
- Motivations: What motivates your child the most?
- Emotional response to stress: What is your child's immediate reaction to a stressor?

In Table 1.2, you can see the characteristics associated with each of these three key areas.

	Activity Level	**Motivations**	**Emotional Response to Stress**
Wood	Superactive	Winning, achieving goals, understanding how something works	Anger, frustration, quick show of temper
Fire	Very active	Being loved, being the star, having fun, understanding what something feels like	Overexcitement, anxiety, mania
Earth	Active, or fluctuates between very active and less active	Pleasing others, being of service, understanding a relationship	Worry, racing or obsessive thoughts
Metal	Enjoys activity and quiet activity	Doing it right, pleasing others, understanding a pattern	Tears, negative thought patterns, fixation
Water	Enjoys activity, but needs alone time	Seeking deeper understanding of why, or what's in it for me, or how I or others benefit	Withdrawal, running away, imagining stories behind the stressor

Table 1.2: Elemental Characteristics in the Three Key Areas

While all the questions in the Five-Element Questionnaire will be helpful in determining your child's Dominant Element, your answers in these three areas are key to understanding your child's Dominant Element. After reviewing the chart, continue reading to learn how to interpret your child's activity level, motivations, and emotional response to stress.

— *"What is my child's activity level?"*

Compared to other children, is your child superactive, active, or active while also liking quiet? Is he active, but needs alone time? Energy levels are most often consistent with a child's Dominant Element as long as the child is healthy and well nourished. You'll need lots of comparisons to determine a child's energy level. If you're tired and rundown, you may feel in the moment that your child is superactive when your child's energy level would be more accurately classified as active.

For example, a Wood child is always busy and on the go until he drops. So, the Wood child probably has school, after-school sports or activities, homework, outside playtime, then finally he collapses in bed when he's completely worn out. In contrast, the Water child is active, but doesn't want to be in a bunch of structured activities. When he gets home, he wants to be alone in his room drawing, reading, or playing with his Legos. He needs alone time to recharge. The trickiest Element to identify is the Earth child because she's smack in the middle with yin and yang qualities. She may be very active and on the go, and then have days where she enjoys some quiet time.

— *"What are my child's motivations?"*

We want to know what makes each child tick. What drives them to act a certain way? Do they want to follow or break the rules? Do they aim to please or do they not really care what others think? That's all under the purview of their motivations.

How children express various traits will vary according to their Dominant Element. For example, every child is curious about the world around him, but a Wood child's curiosity motivates him to explore and figure out things, tending to push the boundaries and touch, feel, and outwardly investigate. On the other end of the continuum, the Metal child is motivated to make order out of chaos by understanding patterns. While the Metal child is extremely curious, he satisfies his curiosity by asking lots of questions, and then he internally reviews the data to determine how something works. The Metal child wants to please his parents and authority figures, so he will tend to figure things out internally rather than push the boundaries.

— *"What is my child's emotional response to stress?"*

When a child is under stress or facing adversity, the emotional reaction to that stress is related to her Dominant Element. Stress can come from not winning a game, not getting her way, a sudden change in plans, or something more serious.

When a Wood child doesn't get her way or loses a game, she easily gets frustrated and angry. If something upsets her, she can lash out verbally or physically to those closest to her, especially her mom. She tends to take things really hard when things don't go as planned, and her parents probably have been working on helping her learn to be a good sport whether she wins or loses.

Now that you understand how to interpret your child's activity level, motivation, and emotional response to stress, review Table 1.2 again. Circle the corresponding characteristics that most closely represent your child's way of being. Is there an element that clearly stands out?

Before moving on to Chapter 2, be sure to take the Five-Element Questionnaire in Appendix A.

Figuring Out My Own Child's Dominant and Influential Elements

I had a difficult time determining my son Nate's Dominant Element. Nate's way of being in the world resonates with both Earth and Fire. He is outgoing, talkative, creative, impulsive, charming, and funny, which are all Fire traits. He's also very loving, helpful, caring, and peacekeeping. He enjoys cooking and eating. He gets very attached to pets, friends, family, and caregivers, which are all Earth traits. At home, I would say that Nate is an Earth child. But in social situations he's more like a Fire child and can sometimes act like the class clown. Before realizing that children have a Dominant and Influential Element, I kept going back and forth between Fire and Earth and had the hardest time trying to decipher which Element he truly was.

After observing him his entire life and paying close attention to his behavior across multiple settings, a few things became clear that helped me figure out his Dominant Element. First, Nate's activity level, while high, is not as high as any of the Fire kids that I know and have worked with. He can sit and read for hours and enjoys some quiet time and being alone on occasion. His activity level resonates with an Earth child more than a Fire child. That was my first clue that Earth may be his Dominant Element. From there I observed his behavior as it related to the two other key areas, motivation and emotional response to stress, and it became clear over time that he resonated with Earth in those key behavioral areas as well.

Ultimately, each child is a unique combination of all Five Elements. Once you understand your child's unique blend of Dominant and Influential Elements, you will be able to understand his behavior, such as what motivates him, how he reacts to adversity, how outgoing he is, how much social interaction he needs, how much physical activity and rest he requires, and how best to parent him to support his Dominant Element.

CHAPTER TWO

Understand and Support Your Unique Child

At this point, you should have a fairly good idea of your child's Dominant Element. If your child is the fullest expression of his element, he was probably pretty easy to classify as you filled out the questionnaire. However, because each child is a unique blend of the Five Elements, you may have only narrowed it down to two or even three elements that describe him. If this is the case, that's totally fine. Reading through this chapter will shed more light on your child's Dominant Element.

As you read about the different elements, you'll gain insight into your child's strengths, challenges, motivations, and physical needs according to his element. Since parenting your child by supporting his Dominant Element is important, I'll conclude each section by exploring ways to understand the emotional expression of each element and offer tips for parenting your unique child to strengthen body, mind, and spirit.

All children have the same basic needs: unconditional love and support, healthy boundaries, good nutrition, physical activity, good sleep, and a stable and secure living environment. However, how we provide these basic needs will vary according to a child's Dominant Element. An Earth child needs affection, cuddling, and verbal reassurance to let her know she's loved, whereas a Water child has less need for physical affection and verbal reassurances. For the Water child, a gentle hand on the shoulder and your loving presence are enough.

Too often in our modern world, we take our children's successes and failures as a reflection of how good a parent we are: If our kids are well behaved and get good grades, that means we're "good" parents, but if our kids are misbehaving in class or struggling to learn, that means we're "bad" parents. Nobody wants to be thought of as good or bad based on external factors that we can't control, but we can release ourselves from this judgment by taking a bird's-eye view of our child's behavior. Rather than take it personally, I've realized that our kids are on their own journey, and their successes or failures aren't always a reflection of our parenting but are part of our journey to learn whatever lessons we're meant to learn.

My experience with Noah really brought this home for me. In the beginning, I felt his eczema reflected my failure as a healer and a parent—a double whammy! But as Noah and I have journeyed through this experience, we've both learned and grown so much. Without the whole experience of Noah's eczema, I wouldn't be in the position I am in and able to write this book right now.

Understanding your child's element and honoring his way of being in the world can take the pressure off both of you to be perfect. When a Water child won't make eye contact or say hi to a stranger, it doesn't mean bad parenting any more than when a Fire child can't stop touching all the breakables in the department store. Instead of being ashamed or annoyed with our kids, we can understand that it's their nature that drives their temperament, and we can help them learn to honor who they are while also finding balance.

Understanding the Wood Child

Strengths

The strength of a Wood child is in his drive to explore, high energy level, and confident demeanor. He has a logical and linear mind. His love of learning shows up as a natural curiosity and inquisitiveness and a desire to figure things out by himself. Hands-on projects, learning, and discovery will engage the Wood child. Enthusiastic and ambitious, he loves to compete and seeks to be first and best at whatever he's into. It is in his nature to continually move forward, push the envelope, overcome challenges, and blaze new trails. His confidence is magnetic, and he attracts many friends; he may lead his social circle. Physically strong and with an abundance of energy, the Wood child often gravitates toward being outdoors, playing sports, and engaging in other physical activities.

Challenges

Because exploration is innate for the Wood child, sitting still or being restrained, whether physically or emotionally, can be particularly difficult for him. When held back or upset about something, he may angrily express his frustration. Logic is how he understands the world, and this can make him impatient and insensitive toward those who don't understand things the way he does. He may talk back, argue, or become defiant when things don't go his way or his ideas or opinions are challenged. In some cases, he may be disrespectful to those in charge and act insubordinately. When he fails to see the logic of why something needs to be done, like homework, he may rush through it so he can move on to what he really wants to do.

Motivations

What motivates the Wood child is figuring things out, setting and achieving goals, and exploring new activities. If you really want to inspire a Wood child, help him with one of his healthy goals. Whether he wants to tie his shoes by himself or save up enough money to buy a toy he desires, talk about and find a way to chart his progress toward his goal. Help him understand the obstacles he may encounter and formulate a plan for overcoming them. This will help lessen his frustration and anger when he faces adversity.

Physical Needs

A Wood child needs plenty of physical activity. Sitting in class all day or playing video games after school can exacerbate the challenges of most Wood children. Encourage outdoor play and exploration time. If you don't live in an area where your Wood child can easily play outside, make sure that weekends are devoted to visiting the park, hiking, or exploring the outdoors in some other way. Exercise, playing outdoors, and being in nature are very balancing for him and give him an outlet for the intense energy he has.

Part of what keeps a Wood child balanced is making sure he's getting enough downtime and sleep. Without adequate rest, a Wood child can actually become hyperactive and impulsive and have difficulty focusing at school. Make sure not to overschedule your Wood child with too many sports or after-school activities and allow him some free time while also encouraging more restful activities, like reading, in the evenings before bed.

Cravings and Addictions

Video games are addicting for most kids, but for the Wood child they can become an obsession. The desire to advance to a new level, earn one more coin, or beat the next opponent can become all-consuming because these things feed the Wood child's innate desire to win. You may need to set very clear boundaries around TV and handheld video games or make them a reward for excellent behavior or the completion of homework and chores.

One of my friends who has a Wood child has banned video games during the week, and her son is allowed to play for only an hour each day on Saturday and Sunday. She says any more game time than that and all he can think about is the next time he'll be allowed to play. He'll ask her 10 times a day when that will be and becomes argumentative and irritable.

Sports drinks, as well as stimulants such as sugar and caffeine, should be avoided. They become very addictive for Wood children and may bring about anger, frustration, irritability, and difficulty sleeping.

Parenting the Wood Child

River is an extremely bright Wood child. He's on the honor roll, and even though he's a grade level ahead of his peers, he doesn't have to work very hard to get good grades. River's mom loves that he never backs away from a challenge, and she is awed by his tenacity in setting and achieving his goals. Because things come easily to River, he takes it extremely hard when he makes mistakes, lashing out verbally and sometimes physically, for instance by kicking a wall. His parents are helping him learn to not dwell on mistakes and to be a good sport. Seeing a counselor has helped him control and release his intense emotions.

For parents of a Wood child, it is important to provide stability and structure and set firm but loving boundaries. Wood children will often test the firmness of the rules, and if enforcement is inconsistent, they can easily use that to their advantage: "You let Timmy have 30 minutes of screen time; why can't I?" They can also be persistent if there's something they want badly, and being vague about whether they can have it may backfire. It's better to make it clear that *no* actually does mean *no*, or that questions are allowed but talking back and arguing are not.

If the Wood child gets irritable, angry, or frustrated by a situation, it's best to help him find an outlet to blow off steam. And even more important, you need to remain calm even when you want to yell back. When River needs to blow off steam, he knows to tell his mom that he needs to go to his room and be alone. Then he'll listen to music or read a book until he's calm and can approach the situation in a better frame of mind.

Wood children also tend to voice their stream of consciousness, which may lead them to seem insensitive or rude. They may even blurt out things that are inappropriate: "Wow! That lady is really old." While it may be true, it's important to help them understand how to frame their thoughts and feelings so they're not hurtful to others. Make sure you're modeling this as well, because Wood children will follow your lead.

Finally, modeling and teaching healthy goal setting and how to work toward achievements are also important for the Wood child. Talking about sportsmanship is a wonderful way of teaching a child how to roll with the flow of winning and losing. It also imparts the lesson that while we can't always control an outcome, we can control how we react to it. Offer constructive criticism, but be careful not be too harsh with your Wood child as that can hurt his pride and spirit.

Understanding the Fire Child

Strengths

Like the sun, the Fire child is magnetic, and those around her like to bask in her glow. In the summer, the sun and its energy are most intense, and there is a veritable delight for the senses— flowers are fully in bloom, the weather is warmer, and colors are richer. It is the same with the Fire child, whose carefree attitude draws others in; she delights in everything around her. She enjoys experiencing new things and exploring her environment with all her senses.

The Fire child is so much fun to be around, and she is usually very comfortable in a variety of social settings. She needs to be with friends and to have plenty of interaction to feel balanced. She enjoys performing in the spotlight and thrives when she has an outlet for her creative side with drama, art, dance, or music.

Things like talking, moving, eating, and thinking may happen fast in the world of a Fire child. She can easily switch her attention from one task to the next, seeking novel experiences that delight the senses. Her lighthearted attitude about life helps keep even serious situations from feeling too heavy.

Challenges

Because she seeks out new and exciting experiences, the Fire child may touch things she shouldn't, because she just can't help herself, or start projects she'll never finish. The Fire child may also become easily bored or distracted. She may constantly need your attention and talk to you with a barrage of "Mom. Mom. Mom. Look at what I can do." She may have trouble finishing her tasks because once she's figured out how to do them, she becomes bored and ready to move on to something more exciting. This can sometimes lead her to be impulsive, doing things without thinking about the consequences first. Her abundance of energy and need for speed and excitement may make her appear hyperactive at times.

While people may think she's thick-skinned, in fact she is very sensitive to what others say and do. Her feelings can easily be hurt, and she can become dramatic when she doesn't get her way or upset when her efforts are not acknowledged. She can have a hard time being serious and sometimes can't stop herself from acting silly, though her bubbly personality will make her well liked by just about everyone.

The Fire child is also sensitive to the energy of other people and is naturally empathetic. Her sensory openness may make her feel more vulnerable to sudden changes in temperature, strong tastes, and loud sounds. She can become easily overwhelmed in places with too much sensory input, such as a crowded mall or amusement park.

Motivations

The Fire child's charisma and charm make her popular with everyone, and she enjoys being the star, feeling adored. Being loved by all is her primary motivation, and she can easily feel rejected if her creative efforts are criticized or ignored.

Physical Needs

To keep a Fire child balanced, you'll need to help her channel her energy and creativity into dancing, singing, sports, acting, or other activities that allow her to explore her creative side.

Because she's in constant motion, you'll need to make sure she regularly eats and drinks throughout the day. She can go from full to intensely hungry in a short span of time, so parents may need to make sure she stops long enough to fill up before she's off on her next pursuit. She may enjoy intense flavors and spicy foods, but she can also be sensitive to changes in flavors. Subtle nuances in flavor are detectable to a Fire child, so she'll know if you've tried to sneak any changes into her regular food. The mom of one of my Fire patients reported that when she tried to add probiotics to her daughter's milk, she refused to drink it.

Just as a fire that burns too brightly can burn itself out, the Fire child needs to balance activity with rest and quiet or she'll get cranky. This may be hard because the Fire child doesn't want to miss out on anything. She may not be able to nap or sleep if there is company at the house or if she feels something is going on without her.

Cravings and Addictions

Refined carbohydrates such as crackers, bread, pasta, and cookies are addictive for most kids, but the Fire child tends to crave them above other foods and may want to limit her diet to mostly carbohydrates. It's important to make sure that she doesn't overdo it on these foods as they offer little nutrition and can affect her blood sugar levels, leading to moodiness and irritability.

Parenting the Fire Child

Harry is a Fire child and is a totally go-with-the-flow, who-cares-if-plans-change kind of kid. He likes to be spontaneous. He's very loving and empathetic and is well liked by teachers and other adults. At the same time, Harry can be demanding; when he wants something, he can get very vocal about it. The hard part is that his high energy level and constant need to talk can be draining for his mom. When she needs a break, she tries to channel his curiosity and energy into more internal pursuits and keeps him busy with myriad art projects.

Because the greatest fear of Fire children is being rejected, you can help yours thrive by offering security, unconditional love, and acceptance. Setting clear boundaries and helping him recognize the difference between appropriate and inappropriate behavior will keep him feeling balanced and in tune with those around him. As a parent, it is important to be calm even when your Fire child is upset or overexcited; this will help him learn to manage his own feelings and energy.

Understand that he's a sensitive kid; although outgoing and charming, he is also easily affected by the emotions of others, especially anger. He is particularly sensitive to being yelled at or talked to with harsh words. While a Fire child can be exhausting at times, it's important not to lash out when he needs your attention. He can easily feel rejected if his efforts to entertain you are met with criticism, and being too harsh with him can have devastating consequences, such as shutting down his creative and lighthearted spirits.

Thinking about others and their needs is also important to model because a Fire kid is easily self-absorbed. Because his thoughts and feelings wash over him quickly, he may not filter what he's thinking and will impulsively blurt out the first thing that comes to mind. He needs to learn to pause before saying things that may be hurtful to others.

The Fire child may try too hard to win the friendship of others, so he needs your help discerning what friendship truly means. His need to be loved and eagerness to please may lead to problems with other children, as he is easily hurt if someone rejects him. It's important to teach him the meaning of true friendship so he doesn't form unhealthy relationships.

Try to use games and play to help make things fun for your Fire child, especially boring chores or homework. You'll also need to help him learn to finish one project before moving on to the next, including putting his toys away before getting out more. Teach him how to be discerning about which projects to start; have him walk through the steps first and consider whether he'll stay engaged until the end. Group activities with a creative aspect will help him channel his need for social stimulation and excitement, as well as aid him in learning to take a project from start to finish.

Most important, make sure to stop and smell the roses, delight in a full moon, or blow on a dandelion with your Fire child. Allow his sense of wonder and joy in the world to wash over you.

Understanding the Earth Child

Strengths

The Earth child is in the middle of the yin-yang continuum and will likely have traits of both yin and yang. At times she will be talkative, silly, charismatic, and outgoing; at other times she'll be quiet and shy until she's warmed up to the situation.

An Earth child will be your friend to the end because relationships are the center of her world. She's very attached to her parents, family, friends, caregivers, teachers, and pets. The Earth child is often described as thoughtful, caring, friendly, trustworthy, and extremely loyal. She's a natural caregiver, helper, or teacher. She may embrace this role very early on in life, showing an affinity for babies and animals, and often being Mommy's or Daddy's helper. She may like to playact being a schoolteacher or mother to her dolls or younger siblings.

The Earth child has a strong connection to food, the bounty of Mother Earth, which is why she enjoys cooking, eating, and sharing her food. She may have an early affinity for cooking and delight in trying new dishes.

According to Dr. Stephen Cowan, author of *Fire Child, Water Child*, Earth children learn through context. In other words, they learn by understanding the connections and relationships among things, which accounts for how mature and well spoken most Earth children are at a young age.[1]

Challenges

While most Earth children are outgoing, talkative, and friendly, they don't necessarily enjoy being the center of attention in social situations. An Earth child may sometimes shy away from performing. In new social situations, she may be quiet and reserved until she makes a friend or finds a way to be useful.

She's able to sort through a lot of information when she understands the context, but when the information confuses her, she is easily overwhelmed, scattered, and disorganized.

Because relationships are foundational to the Earth child, she derives security and sometimes her self-worth from them. She has a tendency to fret over things big and small. When she has a problem, she'll tend to review every possible scenario and solution, but this can lead to obsessive thinking and prevent her from making a decision or taking action.

Since her connection to food is very strong, it's important to set healthy boundaries around food, teaching your Earth child how food nourishes us and provides the basis for energy. When upset or hurt, Earth children tend to comfort themselves with food, possibly leading to overeating. That's why it's important to associate comfort with love and connection instead.

Motivations

What motivates the Earth child is her desire to please others and to lend a hand where needed. As a parent, you can easily get an Earth child to go along with the program if she knows it will make you happy. The downsides are that she may not voice her own needs or desires, and she may be taken advantage of by others.

Physical Needs

It's important to keep the Earth child moving, so make sure she's getting regular exercise. Group sports and activities are usually best because they satisfy her requirements for exercise and her need for community. Without the motivation of seeing friends, she may prefer to get lost in a book or become a couch potato instead.

Cravings and Addictions

Sweets, juice, and refined carbohydrates are particularly appealing to the Earth child, and she can easily overdo it on these foods. If she eats sweets or desserts on a regular basis, she will get into a cycle of craving sweets after meals. In fact, she derives so much pleasure from eating, she can have a hard time limiting herself to a reasonable serving and easily can overeat any food she finds tasty.

Parenting the Earth Child

Scarlett is the fullest expression of an Earth child. She has lots of friends and is a very caring and loving young lady. Friendships can be difficult for Scarlett as her eagerness to please can at times come off as neediness. Her mom is helping her understand that she doesn't need to buy things for her friends or bring them treats for them to like her. When worried about something at school, Scarlett will get a stomachache or become nauseated. This is often resolved when she verbalizes what's upsetting her and her parents can help her find a solution. Talking things out with your Earth child is often very helpful in preventing obsessive or racing thoughts.

To thrive, the Earth child needs to be in a secure and harmonious environment where she feels connected to those around her. She is an affectionate kid who needs reassurance that all is well and that she's loved. Hugs, cuddling, and kisses help fill the need for connection for the younger Earth kid, while an older one will find connection through talking about her thoughts or problems.

The Earth child may feel that her thoughts are not within her control, so it's important to teach her how to handle her thoughts and worries to gain some separation from them. Getting outside or playing with friends is a good distraction. Opening up a line of inquiry such as, "What's the worst that can happen?" can also be helpful in stopping repetitive thoughts. When my Earth son, Nate, gets into a pattern of repetitive thinking, we call it "thought jail," with his thoughts representing the bars. We tell him that he actually has the power to release the bars or let go of those thoughts; he can get out of jail anytime. Sometimes, we actually have him physically act out letting go of the bars and stepping out of jail, which actually helps break his racing thoughts.

Earth children are sensitive to yelling, confrontation, and disagreements. Avoid yelling, fighting, or even punishing another child in front of your Earth child. She'll take what's going on personally, and her worry may lead to stomachaches or digestive problems.

Help your Earth child develop a healthy relationship to food by making sure she eats meals at regular intervals and doesn't snack throughout the day. Try to have meals, especially dinner, at a regular time to avoid hunger that leads to overeating. Make mealtimes social times; encourage talking and storytelling to slow her down. Encourage her to stop eating before she feels full, and if you see she's probably already eaten enough, ask her to wait 20 minutes before having anything else, to allow the sensation of fullness to reach her brain.

It can be really easy to parent an Earth child using food as a motivator. However, rewarding an Earth child with food for good grades, good behavior, or any other reason can set her up for an unhealthy relationship with food as a way to manage her feelings. Make sure to reward your Earth child with praise, affection, and experiences instead of food.

The Fire Child versus the Earth Child

Earth and Fire kids are often the most difficult to tell apart. For one thing, Earth children fall in the middle of the continuum and may have both yin and yang characteristics equally. If you saw this when you took the Yin/Yang Qualities Quiz, chances are you have an Earth child.

In addition, there's a lot of overlap in the way Fire and Earth are expressed through behavior. Both Fire and Earth kids are talkative, sweet, charming, social, and creative. Relationships and family are really important to them.

Let's look at two kids with both Earth and Fire Elements shaping who they are. Note that while there are a lot of similarities between these two girls, their differences in energy level, motivations, and emotional response to stress do set them apart.

Roxy: Earth with a Fire Influence

Roxy is an adorable blonde with rosy cheeks and dimples. I've been working with her since she was nine years old to help resolve her chronic stomachaches and allergies. Even at a young age, Roxy was very well spoken. Now, at age 11, she's outgoing, sweet, and charming, with many friends at school. While Roxy has characteristics of both Earth and Fire, her energy level, motivations, and response to stress are consistent across the board with an Earth child with a Fire influence.

Her energy level is high, but her parents wouldn't describe her as superactive. She loves to read and can spend hours with her nose in a book. This energy level is most resonant with an Earth child.

She's very bright, but she easily gets bored and can tune out, especially with math, her least favorite subject. The annual standardized testing at school causes her a lot of worry; her thoughts race, especially at night. Even though she always does well on her tests, she frets about failing or being held back a grade, which stems from a deep desire to please. Sometimes at school, she doesn't ask for help when she needs it because she's afraid to interrupt the teacher. Her parents must be vigilant to make sure she's getting help when she needs it and must ease her fears about not being good enough.

Roxy's emotional response to stress is worry, which is most closely associated with Earth. When she gets worried, it shows up as digestive complaints like nausea and stomachaches. If she's fighting with her friends, that will also cause her a lot of stress and worry because she wants everyone to get along.

She loves to sing and perform and was even in the talent show at school. Family, friends, and pets are the center of her world, and she's easily swayed to go along with whatever her parents ask of her, if only to keep the peace, which is also most consistent with an Earth child. (In contrast, her Water brother always needs to know "why" before he'll buy into any plan.)

Kacee: Fire with an Earth Influence

Kacee, now age seven, was five years old when I first started treating her for allergies and hives. What I love about Kacee is that she adores cats and always brings her stuffed kitties with her during her treatments. She gives them the most creative names, like Princess Beauty Sprinkle. She has a rich, creative inner world and is always finding a project or craft to entertain herself. She loves to make kitty clothes and accessories and even talks about being a kitty acupuncturist in Kitty World.

Kacee always has a story to tell me and is very outgoing and talkative. Like Roxy, she is charming and articulate, and she has many friends at school. She has a big extended family and enjoys hanging out with her many cousins; family get-togethers are a highlight for her. While all children want to be loved, in typical Fire child fashion, Kacee's desire to be loved and adored by all is highly motivating.

Kacee has more than enough energy to go all day and all night long, which is also consistent with a Fire child. Her parents help her channel it into various creative activities and outdoor play. A natural performer, Kacee was cast in the lead role of her school play, and while she was excited to be the star, she was very anxious about remembering her many lines. Anxiety with fearful thoughts that mentally agitate them is a very common emotional response to stress for Fire kids.

Overall, while Kacee has many Earth traits, her energy level, motivation, and emotional response to stress are all consistent with a Fire child, so she's a Fire child with an Earth influence.

Kacee and Roxy are both articulate, talkative, and charming. They have lots of friends and enjoy family gatherings. They enjoy creative activities and performing. These characteristics are shared by Fire and Earth children.

They differ in their three key areas. Kacee is very active; Roxy is active but enjoys some quiet time. Kacee is motivated by a need to be loved and adored, whereas Roxy is motivated by caring for and pleasing others. Roxy's emotional response to stress is worry with related digestive issues, while Kacee's emotional response to stress is anxiety with fearful thoughts and agitation.

Understanding the Metal Child

Strengths

To a Metal child, life is like one giant puzzle to solve. He sees and understands patterns and identifies details that others overlook. His sharp, perceptive mind is very logical, and he makes sense of things by sorting and organizing data. You'll often find his room tidy, with everything in its place.

His innate quality of discernment allows the Metal child to see the big picture as well as all the little details. When my son Noah, a Metal child, was asked to paint a vase with flowers in art class, he drew not only the vase and the flowers in detail but also the entire background behind it. No other child in the class saw the vase in this same way. This visionary quality is the beauty of the Metal child.

The Metal child has a very strong sense of right and wrong and is very responsible. He understands and respects rules; keeping order and rhythm in his daily routine allows him to know what comes next and makes him feel secure.

Like the Fire child, the Metal child is very sensitive to energy and is naturally empathetic. He may strongly experience or take on the emotions of others, though he may not have the words to express what he's feeling or realize that he's feeling someone else's emotions.

Challenges

When things don't go his way or if he's tired or hungry, the Metal child often gets fixated and becomes inflexible. When he gets upset, tears flow easily. Because he is more sensitive, he can easily become hurt, embarrassed, or frustrated. While normally easygoing, when he's pushed to do something he doesn't want to do or doesn't understand, he has an iron will that can outlast even the most stubborn parents.

When feeling insecure, the Metal child becomes rigid and fixed in the order and routine of the day or in having things go a certain way. If anything is off or different, he may cry, fuss, or complain, and it may be challenging for him to see the situation from someone else's perspective. His desire to get things right and perfect can make him hyper-focused on a task, especially one that he hasn't mastered yet.

The Metal child needs enough downtime to process and discharge all the sensory information he takes in. Otherwise he'll feel overstimulated, which will make it hard for him to settle down for sleep. He may begin to express strong emotions or upsets just before bedtime as the quiet allows them to surface. He'll need your patience and understanding, and your shoulder to cry on, as he releases the feelings that are weighing on him.

Motivations

The Metal child is motivated by doing things right and pleasing those in charge. Unfortunately, this lends itself to perfectionist tendencies. He may be incredibly hard on himself when he makes mistakes. The Metal child may give up easily if he can't master a task or game immediately.

Physical Needs

Being on the yin side of the Five-Element continuum means the Metal child may need more prompting to go play outside. His tightly wound body may be stiffer than other children's; he may have tight hamstrings that make it hard to bend over and touch his toes. Qigong, yoga, and stretching are great ways to keep a Metal child limber.

The Metal child needs to eat meals and snacks at regular intervals. More than any other Element type, he will get so focused on the task or activity at hand that he won't realize he's hungry or thirsty. Only after the first bite does he realize how ravenous he really is.

Cravings and Addictions

The Metal child is very sensitive to tastes and textures. Because he is very discerning and sensitive, he is more likely to be picky about the food he eats. He may crave salty snacks and rich foods.

In addition, video games can be very addicting to the Metal child as his desire to master each level and solve the puzzle can make it difficult for him to disengage from the game. Even if he's no longer playing it, he may continue pondering his next move.

Parenting the Metal Child

At age 13, Kenny is incredibly bright and curious about the world around him. In his reading, logic, and math skills, he is far above the other kids at his grade level. He is very inquisitive and has a strong desire to learn. Routine is very important for Kenny to feel secure. Mom reviews his weekly and daily calendars with him so he knows what his schedule is, who will be picking him up from school, and what after-school activities he has.

He is very sensitive to the environment and the energy of the people around him. His feelings are easily hurt, and he's easily embarrassed by his mistakes. Any slip-up can lead him to have negative thoughts and berate himself for not being good enough. He sees a counselor to help him deal with his feelings and understand how to be more kind to himself.

The Metal child needs consistency and routine to make him feel secure. If he steps out of line, harsh correction will shut him down. Gentle but firm correction and positive reinforcement will work much better for the Metal child. Otherwise, he will get really down on himself and start the negative thought patterns that can lead to depression later in life. In addition, avoid teasing and bringing attention to simple mistakes that don't require correction as this will only frustrate and embarrass the Metal child. It's important to have respect for his sensitive feelings and not intentionally push his buttons.

Don't make idle threats or allow double standards in your parenting. A Metal child has a knack for discernment along with a logical mind, so he'll probably point out any perceived wrongs or inconsistencies in the rules.

It's important to model flexibility to Metal children, so pick your battles carefully. Don't make threats unless you're truly willing to follow through. For instance, don't threaten to keep him at the dinner table until he eats his peas unless you're truly willing to let him sit there all night long. In this case, you might have him lick the peas rather than eat them. Even if you think it would be "giving in," it's best not to engage in a battle of wills that will only leave you both exasperated. This will prevent your Metal child from getting stuck or fixated on perceived wrongs, which is exactly what you're trying to discourage.

Schedule, routine, and rhythm help Metal children adapt to daily life, so give your Metal child as much notice as possible when there's a change in plans. Adequate warning and walking your child through each step of what is going to happen will help him roll with unexpected changes. Going over your schedules daily or weekly is also helpful so he knows what to expect. Discuss different possible scenarios so you can help him approach changes with flexibility.

Understanding the Water Child

Strengths

While reserved and quiet on the outside, the Water child has a deep inner strength and many strong feelings brewing beneath the surface. Don't let her lack of emotional expression fool you into thinking she doesn't care; she keeps her feelings close to her heart. She brings wisdom beyond her years to this life, which is why she's often described as an "old soul." As a master observer, she sees the world differently from others. This wisdom and her powers of observation make a Water child so beautifully innovative and endowed to create in new ways. She will likely enjoy creative and artistic activities in which she can bring the ideas in her head into form.

Her rich inner world is a place she likes to explore, which means she can easily entertain herself and quietly play alone. The Water child will very much go with the flow and can easily transition from one activity to the next as long as you're not rushing her.

Once motivated by something she fancies, she'll pursue it with tenacity. Her courage and quiet inner strength spur her toward her objective—as the river carves out the land, the Water child will move steadily toward her goal.

In social situations, the Water child may be reserved and slow to warm up, but once she feels comfortable, her laid-back nature will come forward. She moves to the beat of her own drum and may not feel the need for a lot of social interaction if her attention is drawn to something that sparks her imagination.

Challenges

The challenge for the Water child is that if she spends too much time in her inner world, she may become disconnected from the people and world around her. She's not readily going to share how she's feeling or what she's thinking, especially when pressured to do so. Because the Water child is more reserved and quiet, she may be out of tune with social nuances. This detachment can leave her feeling like a misfit or left out, which will cause her to retreat further into her own world.

When overwhelmed emotionally, a Water child may become fearful and run away. She may hide under her covers or in a closet, and it is best to give her the space she needs to work through her feelings. Forcing her to talk before she's ready, or asking her to work through a conflict immediately, opposes her natural instinct, which is to let feelings sink in before they are processed. She may not be ready to discuss an upset for a couple of days, so be sure to be patient and give her plenty of time.

Since the Water child marches to the beat of her own drum, she can have difficulty with time management. She can get lost in her own world, easily distracted by something that captures her attention. This leads to difficulty getting ready swiftly when the need arises, such as when trying to get to school and other activities on time.

Motivations

The Water child is motivated by a need to understand the deeper reasons for why something is happening or expected. If the reason for doing something isn't compelling, normal incentives that would excite other element types will not convince a Water child to do what's asked of her. For example, offering to buy her a new toy if she gets 100 percent on a spelling test won't motivate a Water child if she doesn't see why she needs to be a good speller.

Physical Needs

The Water child needs time outside to connect with nature and the world outside her imagination. Find a sport that gets her moving, which will often improve her focus and attention. For Water children who want to connect with their peers, team sports are a great idea. Others will find individual activities such as hiking, golf, or exploring outdoors more enjoyable.

The instinct to retreat within can cause the Water child to disconnect from her physical needs, especially the need to eat and sleep. Having a routine for daily mealtimes, bedtimes, and wake times will help her stay in touch with the needs of her body.

Cravings and Addictions

Salty foods are particularly appealing to the Water child. She may love salty chips, peanuts, and other foods that satisfy this craving. She may also be a meat-and-potatoes kind of kid, refusing to eat vegetables or explore other flavors.

Parenting the Water Child

At age 12, Sandy is incredibly creative and spends hours drawing and sketching. This Water child doesn't feel the passage of time in the same way others do. Her mom gets her up an hour before her brother so she can take her time getting ready for school. Her parents have found it extremely helpful to make sure Sandy has her clothes picked out and her homework in her backpack before going to bed to make the mornings go smoother for everyone.

In nature, Water can take many forms, from a glacier slowly carving out a massive valley to fast-moving rapids smoothing river rocks. Water makes its own way in the world, and in similar fashion, the Water child moves where his imagination takes him. Giving him space to use his own creative imaginations allows him to work through problems in a way that makes sense to him. Honor his approach to problem-solving, even if it seems unusual or foreign to you. Allow him space to complete projects in his own way, even if it differs from yours, provided he's getting the job done and not doing any harm.

A Water child may have difficulty following the constructs of time; there's no rushing the Water child who wants to get ready or eat slowly on his own schedule. Make a fun game of timing activities with your phone or stopwatch.[2] This will help him develop the feeling of how minutes are linked to his daily activities. Also, whenever possible, give your Water child plenty of time to get ready for school or events where punctuality is important.

Just as flowing water turns to unmoving ice, when Water children decide not to do something, it may be difficult to change their minds or motivate them with rewards. You'll find your Water child much more amenable to your requests if you take the time to explain why you want him to do something than if you yell, threaten, or say, "Because I said so."

While all children need affection, love, and reassurance, "less is more" for the Water child. Constant positive feedback and talking can overwhelm him or cause him to retreat. He's often content just being in your presence, which may mean reading in the same room or engaging in other quiet activities like putting together a puzzle or gardening. Just make sure you connect each day, especially at mealtimes. Avoid allowing your child to watch TV or read a book during meals because mealtime is your opportunity to connect and check in with him on a regular and expected basis.

Make sure your Water child has his own private sanctuary he can retreat to when he needs a break. If he is part of a busy family or shares a bedroom, you may need to be a bit creative to make sure he gets the space he needs. If your Water child has siblings who are on the yang end of the continuum, you'll need to pay special attention to make sure he doesn't get left out or become overshadowed by the louder, more demanding siblings.

If you're still not sure which element is dominant in your child, take some time to observe his behavior at home, at school, and in other environments. Pay attention to the three key areas—activity level, motivations, and emotional responses to stress—comparing your child's to those of other children whom you know well. Talk to other parents about their experiences with their kids. I promise that, just as I did with my son Nate, you will figure your child out.

Next we're going to look at the elements in a different way. Just as each element can describe a child's temperament and way of being in the world, it can also relate to the health challenges and illnesses that each child faces. In Chapter 3, I'm going to explain the basics of Five-Element diagnosis so you can understand which problems will arise when an element is out of balance.

CHAPTER THREE

Diagnose Your Child's Imbalances and Health Challenges

You've learned how to use the Five Elements as a tool for understanding who your child is, which will help you nurture and parent your child in a way that is unique to him. Now I'd like to further that knowledge and explain how you can also use the Five Elements as a diagnostic tool to understand the unique health challenges your child faces.

Think of something in your child's health that you feel could be improved. Perhaps your child takes more than an hour to settle down before falling asleep. Maybe he's just had his fifth ear infection and fifth round of antibiotics, and you're leery of another infection. He could be an extremely picky eater who limits his diet to five or six foods despite your best efforts. Or his flaky scalp and extremely dry skin never seem to get enough moisture.

In all these cases, your child is not ill and the doctor can't necessarily fix these problems with a pill, yet something is out of balance. Regardless of the cause, these kinds of challenges are alerting us that something is off. While the issue may resolve on its own over time, it can also persist or even get worse—and if you're like me, hoping your child will outgrow it isn't an option. You want to be proactive now. This is where Traditional Chinese Medicine comes in very handy!

TCM is a wonderful modality for addressing functional problems with no identifiable cause. Rather than focusing on isolating a causative agent such as virus or other pathogen, TCM is concerned with understanding and treating the pattern of imbalance that's creating the symptoms. It looks at what's going on within the context of the whole child.

The way we, as parents, figure out the pattern of imbalance is by understanding the network of functions associated with each of the Five Elements. The Five Elements are interdependent forces that support and regulate one another to achieve balance. When balanced, the Five Elements create health and wellness; when out of balance, health challenges and illness happen. By knowing which element is out of balance, you can write your own healing program to restore health and harmony in your child's body.

For optimal health, we need our qi, or vital force, to be abundant and flowing smoothly throughout the body. We also need all Five Elements to be balanced. Balance is a dynamic process that depends on the quality of our diet, our sleep, our physical activity, and our emotions. When the body is challenged, one or more of the elements will be affected, and the rest of the elements will rise up in support to restore balance. But sometimes, often due to circumstances beyond our control, the body needs a little extra help to regain its balance. That's what this chapter is all about. You will learn how to help your child's body restore elemental harmony.

Five-Element Correspondences for Diagnosis

Just as in nature, we need our personal ecosystem and all Five Elements within it to be balanced for optimal health. For example, a Water imbalance can be created by not drinking enough water, causing our body to become dehydrated. Inadequate water intake, along with exposure to the sun and high temperatures, can cause Fire to blaze out of control in our bodies, which leads to heatstroke. In this way, we can use the Five Elements to comprehend illness.

The Five Elements use a system of correspondences that allow us to understand and contrast the varying aspects of each element (see Table 3.1). In Chapter 2, we focused on the emotional, behavioral, and psychological correspondences related to each element, but in this chapter, we're going to examine the elements as they relate not only to those aspects but also to the physical body and health.

According to Giovanni Maciocia, author of *The Foundations of Chinese Medicine*, "The system of Five-Element correspondences has wide applications in human physiology. . . . Each element encompasses numerous phenomena in the universe and the human body that are somehow 'attributed' to that particular Element. . . . These phenomena 'resonate' at a particular frequency and have particular qualities that respond to a certain Element."[1]

From a physiological perspective, each element corresponds to a set of paired organs, but the way we think of organs is a little bit different in TCM. According to Dr. May Loo, author of *Pediatric Acupuncture*, organs are not viewed as concrete structures with "distinct physical boundaries and attributes," but rather as "energetic organs that have qi channels extending beyond physical entities that are intimately interconnected with each other through Yin-Yang and Five Element relationships."[2]

There is a lot of overlapping vocabulary between Western anatomy and physiology and TCM physiology, but the terms may not always mean the same thing. For instance, when I refer to the Liver and Gallbladder as the paired organs of the Wood Element, I'm talking about the Liver and Gallbladder networks associated with TCM, not the Western view of the liver and gallbladder. As I have just done, I will capitalize the TCM organs to distinguish them from the Western organs.

	Wood	Fire	Earth	Metal	Water
Paired TCM organ networks	Liver and Gallbladder	Heart and Small Intestine	Spleen/ Pancreas and Stomach	Lung and Large Intestine	Kidney and Urinary Bladder
Emotion	Anger	Joy/ Excitement	Worry	Grief	Fear
Western sensory organ	Eyes	Tongue	Mouth/lips	Nose	Ears
Reflected in*	Nails	Complexion	Lips	Body hair	Hair
Tissues	Tendons/ Sinews	Blood Vessels	Muscles	Skin	Bones
Taste**	Sour	Bitter	Sweet	Spicy	Salty
Sound	Shouting	Laughing	Singing	Weeping	Groaning

Table 3.1: Elemental Correspondences in the Body

* "Reflected in" refers to a physical characteristic that indicates the health of a given element and its paired organs. For instance, if a person has nails that easily crack or tear, that person's Wood Element is out of balance.

** Cravings for certain tastes or flavors often indicate imbalances in the corresponding element.

The Wood Element is associated with the TCM Liver network and the Western liver. In TCM, when we say the Liver is the organ corresponding to the Wood Element, it goes beyond our physical liver and into a network of functions associated with the liver and beyond. The Liver nourishes the eyes, playing a role in the eyes' optimal functioning. This functional connection is exemplified in the case of jaundice. When a person gets jaundice from the liver disease hepatitis, it causes the sclera, or white part of the eye, to turn yellow. When you see this color in the eyes, it is a reflection of an imbalance in the Wood Element. There are all kinds of interconnections like this threaded through the Five Elements and TCM functional networks.

In addition to the paired organs, each element corresponds to additional body parts, senses, bodily functions, sounds, odors, tissues, emotions, and so on. How they correspond or connect can't always be directly determined; in such cases, we just have to trust that, in some unknown way, there is resonant energy in the correspondence. However, some of these correspondences align nicely with relationships found in both Chinese and Western medicine. For instance, in TCM there is a correspondence between the Heart and the emotion of joy. Lack of joy, or sadness and depression, creates imbalances in the Fire Element and its corresponding organ, the heart, leading to illnesses like coronary heart disease. In Western medicine there is a large body of research showing that those with coronary heart disease are three times more likely to suffer from depression than the general population.[3]

Once you understand these correspondences, they will help you quickly see which elements may be out of balance in your child. You'll also begin to recognize patterns of symptoms as they develop, and be able to connect seemingly unrelated symptoms with the related element. For example, you may find that when your child's Earth Element is out of balance, she worries, has racing thoughts, and gets stomachaches or loose stools.

Five-Element Sequences for Balance

There's one more aspect of Five-Element diagnosis that is important to understanding your child's pattern of imbalance. It has to do with the interdependent relationships that allow the elements to both generate and regulate one another so no one element gets out of balance.

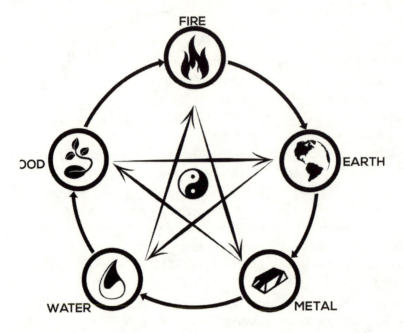

Figure 3.1: Five-Element Chart Sequences

There are two sequences of balance that I'll cover here. The first is the generating, or nurturing, sequence. Looking at Figure 3.1, you can see the circle of arrows moving in a clockwise direction, indicating the generating sequence. Part of each element's role is to feed and nourish the next element in the sequence, going clockwise. For example, in nature, Wood—in the form of trees—provides fuel for Fire. Fires create ash, which feeds and nourishes Earth to produce fertile soil, and so on.

Second, just as each of the elements nurtures and feeds another, they also must regulate and inhibit one another to prevent any one element from getting out of control or becoming excessive. This happens through the regulating sequence. The regulating sequence is represented by the star of arrows in the middle of the diagram in Figure 3.1. In this sequence, each element skips the one next to it and regulates the one after that, preventing that element from getting excessive. For example, in nature, Earth regulates Water by providing boundaries for, say, a river, while Water regulates Fire to prevent it from blazing out of control. In our bodies, the regulating sequence provides a counterbalance so no element grows too great.

In the body when an element is out of balance, mild symptoms will occur at first, but if the imbalance persists, they will progress to a diagnosable illness. By understanding the relationships between the elements and illness, we can understand which elements are out of balance and take measures to restore equilibrium, treat the symptoms, or resolve the illness.

The Causes of Five-Element Imbalance

There are a variety of factors that can create imbalances. For children, the most common factors are:

- Viral or bacterial infection
- Fever
- Too much activity without adequate rest
- Poor sleep
- Poor nutrition
- Dehydration
- Genetic inheritance
- Too much TV, video games, or other mental stimulation
- Stress
- Strong, persistent emotions
- Environment
- Toxins
- Medications

When these factors affect the elements, they can cause elements to be in a state of "excess" or "deficient." Depending on how each element is affected, it will bring about a different set of symptoms. It's common for an element to be in excess at first; if this persists for a long time, the element then becomes deficient, having burned up its qi during the excess phase of imbalance. We need to know whether an element is excessive or deficient to properly restore balance.

An excess element will have more yang qualities such as fever; agitation; loud talking, breathing, or coughing; and thirst. For example, when the Fire Element is excessive, the child may present with facial flushing, loud and fast talking, and restlessness. A deficient element will have more yin qualities such as chills, quiet talking and breathing, weak cough, fatigue, and no thirst. For instance, when the Metal Element is deficient, a child will have cold hands, feet, and nose; a quiet cough; and low immunity. Treatment is different for a deficient versus an excess element. We use herbs and massage to clear heat from the body in the case of the excess Fire Element, but we use herbs and massage with warming and strengthening properties to address the deficient Metal Element.

It's common for a child to have an imbalance in his Dominant and/or Influential Elements. For example, Noah is a Metal child, and his eczema was due to an imbalance in his Metal Element, which also affected his Earth Element. However, I've treated Water kids with Wood imbalances and Fire kids with Metal imbalances. It really just depends on what the underlying cause of the imbalance is.

If a pattern of imbalance persists, it will not affect the original element only; it will often affect the elements along the nurturing sequence as well. Going back to my son Noah's eczema, first his Metal Element was out of balance, which caused dry skin and then eczema. Since Metal was deficient, it started to draw extra nourishment from Earth, which eventually weakened his Earth Element. Eventually this affected the way his body reacted to foods, so he began to have food sensitivities. As both Earth and Metal continued to be out of balance, his symptoms were magnified, and both his issues with food and his eczema worsened.

The other possibility for imbalance lies in the regulating sequence. Let's say a child is really angry. The anger challenges his Wood Element, which becomes excessive. Wood can then overregulate the Earth Element, causing painful gas and digestive problems. So we have to look at the nurturing and regulating sequences as they relate to an imbalance when seeking a diagnosis.

To understand how to use the Five Elements as a diagnostic tool and develop a healing program, we need to first look at each elemental network and its related activities and responsibilities in the body. Then we'll go over the types of symptoms that occur when each element is out of balance and is either excessive or deficient. (Some symptoms will sound very similar, but represent different diagnoses in TCM.) The three main areas that will be addressed for each element are psychological, physical, and emotional imbalances. Then, in the next chapter, I will walk you through the general treatment plan I use with the patients in my clinic and show you how to customize it to fit your child's individual needs, based on his Elemental imbalances.

The Functions of Wood

In TCM, the Wood Element is responsible for the flow of qi throughout the body, which influences our digestion and ability to properly secrete bile. Because our qi is connected to our emotions, the Wood Element is also responsible for the smooth flow of our emotions. It's normal for our emotions to vary throughout the day or week. When Wood is in balance, we can easily move through our emotions and not get stuck or fixated on any particular one. When the Wood Element becomes excessive, it can cause easy frustration and irritability or magnify other emotions we're experiencing.

The emotion associated with the Wood Element is anger, which is sure to make itself known at various levels when Wood is out of balance. If emotions—especially anger—are repressed for a long period, it can lead to depression as well. Wood is also the first element directly affected by stress.

The paired organs associated with the Wood Element are the Liver and Gallbladder networks. The Gallbladder network, as with the Western gallbladder, secretes bile, which helps the body digest fats. Eating too many fatty foods can be taxing on the Wood Element. The Liver network is responsible for storing our blood and regulating our blood and fluid volume. In women, it also regulates menstruation. That's why many women feel heightened emotions and irritability around their period if their Wood Element is excessive. If deficient, women might experience fatigue around their menses. If teenage girls have menstrual issues such as cramping, irritability, breast tenderness, or an irregular cycle, it is likely they have a Wood imbalance. In my experience, intervening early with acupuncture and herbal medicine, rather than merely managing symptoms with pain medicine or birth control pills, can prevent lifelong menstrual issues.

The Wood Element connects with the eyes and governs the sinews, or tendons and ligaments.

April is a Water child whose Influential Element is Wood. When April was younger, she had difficulty managing her emotions, particularly anger and frustration. Like many children who have Wood as their Dominant or Influential Element, she has a quick temper. But for April it was more than that; she had an imbalance in her Wood Element. She could keep it together at school, but at home she would lash out verbally, particularly at her mother, using mean and hurtful words—a sign of an excessive Wood Element.

With the help of a family counselor, April's parents taught her to express her strong emotions by writing them in a notebook. The pause to write them down instead of saying them in the heat of the moment gave April the space she needed to get a handle on her emotions and process what she was feeling. April now recognizes when she's overstimulated and goes to her room to be alone, which helps her find her inner calm.

April's treatment plan included monthly acupuncture, going to bed early enough to get adequate sleep, eating meals at regular intervals, avoiding sugar and processed foods, and getting plenty of physical activity. The combination has helped rebalance her Wood Element. Now, at age 11, she recognizes that physical activity, like playing her favorite sport of softball, and eating before she's starving will help balance her moods so she can feel positive and healthy.

Wood Imbalances

When a person is always on the go, the energy of the Wood Element won't be properly nourished by Water and can eventually become depleted. Things like not eating, eating on the run, or grabbing junk food snacks in order to move on to the next thing will eventually catch up with the body, especially the Wood Element. When the Wood Element is out of balance, you will see one or more of the following physical symptoms in your child, depending on whether Wood is excess or deficient.

Deficient Wood	Excess Wood
Fatigue	Headaches, especially at the temples or top of head
Eyestrain	
Blurry vision	Migraines
Insomnia, difficulty falling asleep, or light sleeping	Muscle spasms
	Red, irritated eyes
Environmental or food allergies	Restlessness, difficulty sitting still
Food intolerances and difficulty digesting gluten/dairy	
	Heartburn, ulcers
Depression with anger and frustration	Uncomfortable or foul-smelling gas
	Oily, acne-prone skin

Table 3.2: Physical Symptoms of Imbalanced Wood

Jake is a Wood child who, when his Dominant Element is excessive, is what some people would call "a handful." He is incredibly active all day and then crashes at night. His mom can always tell when he needs more sleep or has eaten too much sugar because he can't stay in one place and complains of a headache. At those times, he will exhibit incredible defiance and anger toward his parents and others because he can't seem to get himself under control.

Jake's treatment plan included avoiding sugar and processed foods, taking herbs to balance his excess Wood Element, adding probiotics, and focusing on good-quality fats. In addition, we added acupressure at home for balancing the Wood Element. This has helped him reduce his headaches and balance his energy and emotions.

In-Balance Psychological State	Out-of-Balance Psychological Issues
Curious, exploring, goal-driven, ambitious, confident, energetic, athletic, strong	Hyperactive, out-of-control, impulsive, insubordinate, argumentative, insensitive, impatient, defiant, depressed

Table 3.3: Psychological Manifestations of Wood

When the Wood Element is out of balance, either excessive or deficient, this may show up emotionally as bouts of anger, frustration, or in extreme cases defiance, rage, and physically lashing out.

The Functions of Fire

The Fire Element is associated with the most important of the TCM organ networks, the Heart and Small Intestine. In TCM, the

Heart network is viewed as the "emperor" of the body, ruling over physical, emotional, and spiritual well-being.[4] The Heart network, like the Western heart, moves the blood in the blood vessels and is responsible for its smooth flow, which is essential for our immediate survival. The Heart network is paired with the Small Intestine network, which has the job of separating pure from impure as it relates to digesting food. However, the Small Intestine also has a role in our psychological well-being. It helps us sort our experiences in a similar way, allowing us to make decisions and understand right from wrong. When this aspect of the Fire Element is out of balance, a child may have difficulty making wise choices or following the rules because right and wrong are not readily apparent.

The most important aspect of the Fire Element is that the Heart network houses the *shen,* or spirit and mind. When our Fire Element is balanced, the mind is calm and communication is easy. Our creativity and passion pour through, allowing us to experience love, joy, fun, happiness, and contentment. However, when the Fire Element is out of balance, thoughts become disordered. Anxiety, restlessness, speech issues, and difficulty focusing and remembering can occur. Tempers flare and moods change easily as Fire flares or blazes out of control. When the Fire Element is out of balance over a long period, severe emotional and psychological issues can arise.

The Fire Element is associated with the tongue, which is why issues related to speech will arise when Fire is out of balance. Because Fire is responsible for the flow of blood, the health of this element is also reflected in one's complexion. A healthy, rosy complexion with luster indicates balanced Fire, whereas a dull or pale complexion indicates a deficient Fire Element.

Sam is an Earth child with a Fire influence. He's funny, charming, and a bit of a chatterbox. When his Fire Element is deficient, Sam gets easily distracted, forgetting simple tasks he's just been asked to do, such as putting his dishes in the dishwasher. His mom has to remind him several times to complete these tasks, and his parents have to sit with him the entire time he's doing his homework to keep him focused. If they don't, it can take him almost two hours to finish work that should take only 30 minutes. Sam's treatment plan included making sure he goes to bed early enough to get enough sleep, acupuncture and herbs to treat the deficient Fire network, and at-home acupressure and massage.

Fire Imbalances

When the Fire Element is excessive, it's like a flame burning too brightly. Our minds and spirits become restless and ungrounded, and the emotional and psychological well-being of a child suffers. When the Fire Element is deficient, it's like the last, smoldering embers of a fire breaking down.

Deficient Fire	Excess Fire
Tendency to tire easily, lack of stamina	Overexcitement
Lack of focus, distractibility	Anxiety, panic, fears
Feelings of being scattered or overwhelmed	Flushing, red face, sweating
Mental and emotional disorders	Sores on mouth, lips, or tongue
Forgetfulness	Rashes, hives
Light sleep, easily woken by ambient sounds	Speech problems such as stuttering, difficulty articulating
Excessive sweating, spontaneous sweating	Insomnia, excessive dreaming, nightmares, restless sleep
Fear of rejection, phobias	Mood swings, quick-temperedness
Need for adoration and friendship	Inability to think straight, tendency to be overwhelmed, difficulty making decisions

Table 3.4: Physical Symptoms of Imbalanced Fire

Kandace is a sensitive Fire child with a Metal influence. When she was very young, her parents divorced, and her mom worked full-time while raising her. Since there wasn't enough money for regular child care, Kandace was shuffled around to various friends' houses after school until her mom returned from work. Kandace felt very insecure, not knowing how her week would unfold or who would be watching her while her mom worked. To add to her unstable home life, when she was with her dad (a Wood type), he would yell and scold her if she did anything wrong or touched something she shouldn't have. This caused Kandace to retreat inward and experience racing thoughts and anxiety because her Fire Element was excessive. Eventually Kandace began to have an extremely hard time going to sleep, and she would toss and turn and wake up several times each night with nightmares, which led to her being tired and unfocused at school.

When I first saw Kandace to work on her sleeping issues, she was very shy and quiet. I'd notice her quietly exploring my office, tentatively reaching out to touch something. The first step in her healing program was to help her parents recognize that their daughter was a sensitive Fire child who needed stability. Because her Influential Element was Metal, she needed more rhythm and routine in her weekly schedule. Her mom was able to arrange for Kandace to regularly spend the afternoons at her best friend's house. We then put a nighttime routine in place to help her unwind from the day. In addition to regular acupuncture treatments to nourish Kandace's Fire Element, we used herbal medicine and massage after her bath, along with a guided meditation with progressive relaxation to help quiet her mind before bed.

As Kandace got more rest and her home life became more stable and secure, she began to come out of her shell, eventually taking an interest in drama and acting. Now in junior high school, she understands that her sensitive nature came from her dominant Fire Element, and she is relieved to know that there isn't anything "wrong" with her. She knows that she's been gifted with sensitivity, passion, and creativity, which she now pours into her favorite after-school activity, drama club.

In-Balance Psychological State	Out-of-Balance Psychological Issues
Creative, engaging, charismatic, sensation-seeking	Dramatic, impulsive, loud, silly, obnoxious, discourteous, manic, anxious, panicky, phobic, moody, quick-tempered, hyperactive, impulsive

Table 3.5: Psychological Manifestations of Fire

The emotion corresponding to the Fire Element is joy, but as with all other emotions we're not meant to stay in a constant state of joy. Too much of it can manifest as overexcitement, which can morph into anxiety, panic attacks, and even mania.

The Functions of Earth

The main functions of the Earth Element are to break down and digest the food we eat, and then to distribute the resulting nutrients around the body to every organ, tissue, and cell. In TCM, this digestive function is referred to as transforming and transporting food essence, and the organ network is known as the Spleen and Stomach network. (The Spleen network would be more aptly called the Spleen/Pancreas network because its functions are closely associated with the functions of those two Western organs.) The Stomach network receives the food and the Spleen/Pancreas network digests it, transforming it into qi and blood. As the Earth Element relates to digestion, it is fitting that it's also associated with the mouth, lips, and secretion of saliva, all essential to the first steps in digestion. When the Earth Element is out of balance, the first signs—such as stomachaches, nausea, loose stools, constipation, gas, or bloating—are often related to digestion.

The Earth Element controls the blood to the extent that it transforms the nutrients from our food and turns them into blood to nourish the body. It also controls the blood by keeping it secured in the blood vessels, which avoids hemorrhaging or excessive menstrual bleeding. The health of the Earth Element is reflected in the muscles, particularly in our arms and legs. When the transforming and transporting functions are working properly, we'll have strong muscles, but if not, our muscles will be weak and easily atrophy. Fatigue, especially chronic fatigue, is most often a sign of an Earth imbalance. When the Earth Element is balanced, we'll have adequate blood traveling throughout our bodies, we'll be well nourished, and we'll have plenty of energy, good digestion, and strong muscles.

The Earth Element houses the intellect, or *yi* in TCM. Our intellect allows us to study, learn, memorize, sort data, and problem solve. It helps us focus, concentrate, and generate ideas. When the Earth Element is out of balance, there may be slow thinking, difficulty remembering, and an inability to focus on one's studies. Overstudying and overworking greatly affect the Earth Element.

Gemma is an Earth child with a Fire influence, and she is a sweet, kind, loving young lady. With Earth being her Dominant Element, she tends toward worry, which can easily cause her Earth element to become excessive. Her main worries are about homework and friends. She's always been prone to nausea, stomachaches, and loose stools, which are aggravated by her intense worries.

When I started treating Gemma, our first action was to eliminate food chemicals, and we discovered that artificial colors, flavors, and preservatives, especially monosodium glutamate (MSG), were big triggers. Food-sensitivity testing later showed that sugar and gluten were also triggers. When we tracked Gemma's food intake over a school week, it was eye opening to see how high her sugar intake really was. With nightly desserts, treats at school, and the occasional soda, she was ingesting upwards of 60 grams of sugar on some days. Her nightly desserts were escalating Gemma's digestive upsets and her worries. Eliminating refined sugar and artificial colors, flavors, and preservatives helped with her stomachaches and nausea and calmed her worries considerably.

Now when Gemma worries, she's able to put things in perspective by doing an internal inquiry. Is this something she really needs to worry about? Is there anything she can do right now to solve the problem or at least make herself feel better? Sometimes it helps allay her worry to realize that the worst-case scenario isn't likely to happen, and even if it does, she can handle it. If this doesn't help, then it's time for distraction. To take her mind off her worries, Gemma likes to hang out with a friend and draw or read a book. We also have Gemma take flower essences, like Bach Rescue Remedy, when she's feeling really worried.

Earth Imbalances

When the Earth Element is out of balance, a child will present with one or more of the following physical symptoms depending on whether Earth is deficient or excessive:

Deficient Earth	Excess Earth
Digestive problems, especially gas, bloating, constipation	Constant hunger, overeating
Recurrent abdominal pain or stomach upset, ulcers	Craving for sweets after meals
Low or high blood sugar	Tooth decay
Overweight, obesity	Soft muscles or poor muscle tone
Emotional eating, overeating	Sugar cravings
Thick mucus in sinuses	Tendency to tire easily, lack of stamina
Headache with heavy feeling, or related to worry or conflict	Loose stools or diarrhea
Weak joints	Nervous stomach leading to urgent bowel movements
Fatigue, difficulty getting started	Food allergies, sensitivities, or intolerances

Table 3.6: Physical Symptoms of Imbalanced Earth

Damian is a Water child with a Metal influence. He's allergic to peanuts and eggs, and if he eats either one he begins to vomit. Dairy and bananas were also a problem for him, causing eczema and loose stools. These symptoms were due to an imbalance in his Earth Element. Eventually this started affecting his Metal Element, causing skin issues such as dryness and eczema.

To help Damian heal, it was important for his parents and all of his caregivers to avoid giving him dairy and bananas. It was hard for Damian's parents to get his grandparents—who watched him several nights a week—to understand why he couldn't have dairy. His grandparents thought it unwise to avoid it and were sneaking it into his diet despite his parents' wishes. Once his grandparents finally understood the importance of removing dairy from his diet, Damian's loose stools resolved. The eczema was significantly better after just three weeks, and by week six it was almost completely healed.

In-Balance Psychological State	Out-of-Balance Psychological Issues
Caring, helpful, thoughtful, able to work well with others, plenty of energy, clear thinking, good memory	Low self-esteem, insecure, needy, disorganized, overwhelmed, separation anxiety, not voicing needs, racing thoughts

Table 3.7: Psychological Manifestations of Earth

Worry is the emotion associated with the Earth Element. Earth children tend toward worry and its more extreme version, obsessive thinking. Because of an Earth child's innate desire to maintain peace and harmony and keep everyone happy, she will worry about things big and small in her world; anything that might threaten peace and harmony will be food for her mind to ruminate on. This may then affect her digestion and sleep if left unchecked.

The Functions of Metal

The Metal Element is associated with the Lung and Large Intestine networks. The most important function of the Lung network is respiration and breathing. As mentioned in Chapter 1, there are many forms of qi. In TCM terms, respiration represents the inhalation of clean qi, or oxygen, and the exhalation of dirty qi, or carbon dioxide. In addition, the Lung network is in charge of dispersing the qi we think of as our vital force throughout the body. The Lung network also works closely with the Heart network to help control blood circulation, as the qi leads the blood, circulating it around the entire body. Thus, when the Lung network is strong, the chest is open, breathing is easy, and qi and Blood flow smoothly.

The Lung network is associated with the skin, which is also thought to "breathe" and is in direct contact with the outside environment. It acts as a protective barrier between the body and environment and is part of our defense system. The Lung network controls the space between the skin and the muscles, where another manifestation of qi, called the defensive qi, or *wei qi*, resides. Our defensive qi protects us from external pathogens such as toxins, viruses, bacteria, and fungi. It also controls sweating and the proper opening and closing of our pores to regulate our body temperature, and it warms the skin and acupuncture meridians. When the Metal Element is in balance, our immune system is strong; our body can resist illness and recover in a timely manner.

The Lung network is said to help regulate fluid balance in the body, keeping the skin, tissues, and membranes properly moistened. Another aspect of fluid regulation comes from the Large Intestine network, which pulls water back into the body to help with fluid regulation, further separating pure from impure and excreting waste from the body.

The Western organs associated with Metal are the nose and throat, and Metal also controls nasal mucus. When the Metal Element is in balance, the skin will be properly moistened, the nose clear, and the voice strong.

Ben is a Metal child with a Wood influence. He's incredibly bright and articulate, and his cognitive abilities are far ahead of his peers'. What troubles Ben is that he's highly sensitive emotionally and incredibly hard on himself if he doesn't complete a task well. During the day he seems fine, but at night before bed the negative thought spirals begin. He can't stop thinking about all the things that he did wrong that day. When his Metal Element is excessive, he has really negative self-talk and tells himself he's an idiot. As his thoughts spiral out of control, he feels like he's the worst person in the world with no friends and no life. As these strong emotions build up, his excess Metal overregulates Wood, and he begins to feel angry and depressed.

Once Ben's parents realized they could no longer reassure or console him, they brought him to my clinic. We started with an elimination diet and discovered he was extremely sensitive to gluten and dairy. Ben's depressed mood improved dramatically after we eliminated them. In addition, his parents removed artificial colors, flavors, and preservatives from his diet and added glutamine and probiotics. He now has regular acupuncture treatments and herbs to balance his Metal and Wood Elements, along with acupressure at home. Most important, understanding that he's a sensitive Metal child has helped his parents be more compassionate about his sensitivity and recognize that what seems like an exaggeration is really how he's feeling. It has also allowed Ben to express his feelings to his parents without being disregarded.

Metal Imbalances

When the Metal Element is out of balance, a child will present with one or more of the following physical symptoms, depending on whether Metal is excess or deficient:

Deficient Metal	Excess Metal
Congested nose and sinuses	Stiff muscles, lack of flexibility
Chronic food and environmental allergies	Hypersensitivity to taste, touch, smell, and sound
Colds that rapidly go to the chest	Easily triggered gag reflex
Frequent illness or upper respiratory tract infections	Dry skin, hair, nails
	Eczema
Chronic runny nose	Chronic stuffy nose
Chronic eczema and/or psoriasis	Shortness of breath
Chronic irritable bowel syndrome	Cough, croup, stridor
	Asthma
Tendency toward infections— sinus, skin, nose, chest	Allergies
	Sinus problems
Sensory processing disorders	Ear infections
	Constipation with dry stools

Table 3.8: Physical Symptoms of Imbalanced Metal

Gary is a Fire child with a Metal imbalance that clearly placed him in the unwellness gap. When Gary's parents first brought him in for treatment, he was sick more often than he was well. He had repeated ear infections, croup, and a perpetually runny nose. In addition, his growth had slowed, and his doctor was concerned about his lack of weight gain. This indicated that his Earth and Water Elements were also being affected.

Gary's parents were looking for a better way to deal with their son's state of chronic unwellness, frustrated with all the rounds of antibiotics and resorting to feeding him ice cream to help him gain weight. We started by eliminating dairy from his diet. While his parents were reluctant at first, after the two-week elimination trial his chronic runny nose was gone, and it returned only if he ate dairy again.

In addition, we started a regimen of acupuncture, at-home daily massage, and herbal medicine, and we added glutamine, fermented foods, and probiotics to his diet. It took about six months to rebalance his Metal Element, strengthen his immunity, and help his body heal on its own without intervening with antibiotics. Most important, we restored his and his parents' trust that his body could heal on its own without medication.

In-Balance Psychological State	Out-of-Balance Psychological Issues
Discerning, well-behaved, loyal, strong sense of right and wrong, thrives on routine, particular, organized	Inflexible, resistant to change, obsessed with order or routine, low self-confidence or self-esteem, deeply wounded by criticism, perfectionist, fear of doing things wrong, negative, spiraling negative thinking

Table 3.9: Psychological Manifestations of Metal

The emotions that have the most impact on the Metal Element are sadness and grief. A Metal child may easily cry when feeling strong emotions of any kind, including happiness or joy. This can be particularly hard on boys, whose tendency to tears may lead to teasing and name calling. Metal children are highly sensitive to just about everything: emotions, taste, touch, smell, and sound. It can be difficult to understand how Metal children see the world, but trust that when they tell you something, what they're expressing is truly how they feel and not just an exaggeration.

The Functions of Water

The TCM organ networks associated with the Water Element are the Kidney and Urinary Bladder. The most important aspect of the Kidney network is its role in directing our birth, growth, and development. It also governs reproduction as children go through puberty and then reach reproductive maturity, eventually passing their genetic inheritance to their children. In addition, the Kidney network governs water and other fluids in the body. It also works closely with the Earth Element, providing the digestive fire for the Spleen/Pancreas network to perform its transforming and transporting functions. The Water Element also controls the bones and is associated with the ears. When the Water Element is balanced, our children grow and develop at a normal rate and meet their developmental milestones on time. When Water is out of balance, there will be issues related to the bladder, bones, teeth, and ears.

When the concepts of TCM were being formed, the workings of the brain and nervous system had not yet been elucidated; however, the functions related to the brain and nervous system were presumed to be associated with the Water Element. At that time, it was understood that eating fat supported brain and spinal cord function, and as we know today, cholesterol is essential to healthy brain function. When the Water Element is strong and balanced, a person will have normal cognition, memory, and concentration.

Divya was 22 months old and still not walking. She would hold on to the coffee table and stand up, but upon letting go she didn't have the strength to stay standing without help. In addition, she had very few words, saying only *mama* and *ball*. On top of speech, occupational, and physical therapy, Divya's parents brought her to my clinic to get extra support because she wasn't progressing very quickly with her other therapies. Failing to meet her developmental milestone of walking, her lack of age-appropriate speech, and her slightly low muscle tone pointed to deficient Water, Fire, and Earth Elements. In order to support these deficient elements, we used a combination of scalp acupuncture, *tuina* massage, and acupressure at home. To support all three elements, she was prescribed extra fish oil, foods with omega-3 fatty acids, bone broth, and herbs. Within just a few weeks, Divya began to progress more quickly, and within a couple of months she began to try her first steps.

Water Imbalances

When the Water Element is out of balance, a child will present with one or more of the following physical symptoms, depending on whether Water is excess or deficient:

Excess Water	Deficient Water
Dry nose and throat	Lack of focus, poor memory and retention
Difficulty falling asleep	Cold hands and feet
Fears or phobias, especially fear of the dark	Tendency to easily tire out, low stamina
Bladder infections	Bedwetting
Kidney stones	Delayed milestones
Hypersensitivity to light and loud sound	Cavities, poor bone or tooth development
Coarse or brittle hair	Backache or knee pain
Tendency to be easily frightened	Delayed closure of the fontanelle
	Hearing problems
	Genetic conditions (all)
	Cognitive impairment

Table 3.10: Physical Symptoms of Imbalanced Water

Water child Chris is quiet with a dry, quirky sense of humor. He's incredibly bright, but his grades were poor because he had trouble paying attention in class. He would do his homework, then forget to turn it in. His parents tried all kinds of reward systems, but not much seemed to motivate Chris. Some of his teachers thought he was lazy and doing the minimum to get by. His parents worried that he was depressed and were constantly on him about his grades and his behavior. They put him in structured activities after school, which didn't seem to help. Whenever they tried to talk to Chris about all of this, he'd just look at them stoically and shut down, retreating further into his inner world.

Chris had a deficient Water Element. To balance his Water Element, we started regular acupuncture treatments and herbs as well as simple lifestyle changes. We helped his parents understand that less is more for the Water child, so they curbed the excessive talking, yelling, and attention given to his grades. What he needed was *some* structure and routine, but also time to be alone to explore his inner creative urges.

To help Chris find his motivation, we worked on getting him some momentum, which started with adding movement in his daily routine. He started on the swim team and found it to be a great way to help him be more active and connect with other kids. His parents also got him involved in the card game *Magic: The Gathering*, and he found a group of friends with whom he feels like he belongs. As his parents gave him more space in his schedule and stopped pressuring him, it helped him come back into balance, thereby finding the motivation to start getting better grades.

In-Balance Psychological State	Out-of-Balance Psychological Issues
Wise, imaginative, inner strength, goes with the flow, easygoing, emotionally intelligent	Depression, lack of appropriate fear, numerous fears/phobias, unmotivated, withdrawn, silent, stoic, absentminded, lack of confidence, lack of trust in others, gloomy, melancholic

Table 3.11: Psychological Manifestations of Water

The emotion associated with the Water Element is fear, and children with an imbalance in their Water Element will have fears and phobias that stop them from doing certain activities. Water children are particularly prone to being easily frightened. Water is said to be the source of willpower, or *zhi*. Our Water Element gives us courage and helps us find the will to move through the ups and downs of life and tenaciously pursue our goals.

Figure Out Your Child's Elemental Imbalances

Now that you have a sense for the role each element plays in your child's health, it's time to figure out which elements are out of balance for your child. Take the Five-Element Diagnostic Test in Appendix B or at www.robinraygreen.com/healyourchild.

Keep in mind that you're not looking just to diagnose illness, but to see all the big and small things that are affecting your child's body, mind, and spirit. Remember that when one element is out of balance, others will also be affected, so it's okay to see symptoms in your child that correspond to more than one element. This test will help you find the pattern of imbalance creating disharmony in your child's body and determine which element or elements are most in need of rebalancing.

With a better understanding of your whole child, you can now use the following chapters to learn a general approach to supporting your child's health and create an individual healing program.

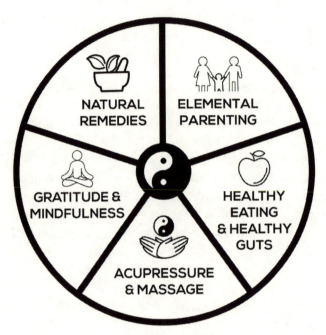

The Wellness Wheel

CHAPTER FOUR

Heal Your
Whole Child

It is now time to start developing your child's individual healing program. Bringing the elements back into balance is sometimes fairly easy, especially when it comes to acute conditions such as a minor head cold. But for chronic conditions or recalcitrant problems, it is a gradual process that can take time. There isn't a quick fix.

Whether your child is suffering from a mild imbalance or a severe health condition, the best advice I can give you is to surrender to the fact that "it is what it is." I'm not saying that you should be apathetic or give up. Instead, by detaching from the situation, you can realize that the symptoms are pointing you in the direction of what truly needs to be addressed. The imbalance is actually telling you what needs to be healed and inspiring action to support healing. We can see our children's suffering as an opportunity for change and growth not only for our children, but for ourselves and the rest of our family.

No matter what, bringing the elements back into balance starts with the same general approach. It begins by addressing issues in five areas of focus that make up what I like to call "The Wellness Wheel": elemental parenting, acupressure and massage, healthy eating and healthy guts, natural remedies, and gratitude and mindfulness.

- *Elemental parenting* means consciously creating a lifestyle that supports your child's unique Five-Element type and along with it a harmonious family life. It means taking full responsibility for the fundamentals every kid needs—love, food, sleep, and movement in just the right amounts.
- *Acupressure and massage* both promote wellness and treat illness. Making them a part of your daily routine will have a positive impact on your child's health, and they can be used in conjunction with Western medical treatments.
- *Healthy eating and healthy guts* are the foundation of optimal physical health and proper growth and development.
- *Natural remedies* refers not only to things like herbs, homeopathic medicines, and acupuncture, but also to having a healthy, nontoxic home. While I don't cover specific remedies in this book, I'll recommend resources to help you pick the right ones.
- *Gratitude and mindfulness* are habits that we want to instill in our children to help create appreciative and happy kids who are resilient when they face stress or adversity.

This chapter is intended to give you an overview of all the areas that can be addressed to help your child achieve balance. It's here to give you a framework to use in writing your child's individual healing program. You don't need to implement all the changes at once or even follow all the recommendations. They are intended to spark ideas and help you tune in to all the forms of medicine that are readily available to you and your child.

These recommendations broaden the definition of *medicine* to include more than drugs. Medicine is found in many different forms, from a kind word, a hug, a plant, or a massage to a quiet place to think or be in nature. These are *all* forms of medicine, and there's little to no cost for many of them.

Remember, this is a healing journey, and it will take time. Lean into it. Start gradually with the easiest things first, and then add more one by one. Go gently on yourself. You may find yourself thinking, *If only I'd known this sooner or done that differently.* You didn't know what you didn't know. That's okay. You're starting today, and the fact that you're reading this book right now means you're already on the path to healing your whole child—and that's the most important thing. Holding on to guilt about what you did or didn't do in the past will not help you or your child. It's time to let it go and move forward.

Under each category, there will be general advice that applies to all elemental imbalances. Certain element types may have challenges in some categories, and I've added specific advice for these cases. As you read through this chapter, I urge you to take notes and underline the actions that would be easiest for you to implement right now. You can organize the steps that are most important by going to the template in Appendix C and starting to fill out your child's individual healing program. You'll want to continuously fill in the template in Appendix C as you read through this book, rather than trying to fill it all out at once. The chapters that follow will provide even more in-depth information on how to improve your child's diet as well as how to achieve balance with acupressure and massage.

Elemental Parenting

With elemental parenting, the intention is to support our children and honor their Dominant Element, as well as to create a harmonious family life. Ultimately it's up to us to make sure that our children's fundamental needs are met. Every child needs to be loved and to eat, sleep, and move. When these fundamental needs are not being met, it is sure to create elemental imbalances and eventually illness. Elemental parenting requires us to do some self-reflection and become a better version of ourselves so we can model the attitudes, habits, and fundamentals that we want to cultivate in our children. To do this, we must understand our own elemental makeup and imbalances.

As you read through and determined your child's Dominant Element, you also probably figured out your own. You may find that this information explains the differences or similarities that you have with your child. As you write down ideas for your child's healing program, it's also important to evaluate yourself and your role in contributing to your child's health challenge. What do *you* need to change? Do you need to alter the language you're using? Do you need to model more flexibility for your Metal child or calmness for your Fire child? Are you overscheduling yourself? Do you get enough sleep? Do you balance rest and activity? Are you addicted to carbohydrates or processed foods? We can't expect our kids to act differently from how we act, so it's important for us to address issues that affect our own health and then our children's health.

My best friend, Kelly (a Fire type), realized that she needed to be calmer and less reactive when dealing with her son (a Wood type). When he's upset about something, he's quick-tempered and can start shouting, which can flare Kelly's Fire nature and make her want to snap or yell back. But she quickly realized this just escalated the situation. To support her son, she has started practicing daily meditation so she can be calmer in heated situations. This has even helped balance her Fire Element. We teach our children, but our children are also the teachers of some of the biggest lessons we have to learn.

As parents, we also bring our own history and experience into how we parent and relate to our children. Our fears, doubts, and worries can affect our kids. It's not what we say, it's what we do that has the most impact. For instance, if we have a fear of germs and getting sick, our actions in relation to these areas will affect our children. If we're constantly washing our hands and afraid of touching a doorknob or shopping cart, our kids will absorb these fears, too.

How we talk to our kids and the words that we use are also very important. Without realizing it, we can impart subconscious, self-sabotaging ideas in their young minds. If a child is frequently ill, you might be tempted to say, "He's always sick." If a child has high energy, you might quip, "She's got ADHD." Similarly, if your child is sick, you might say, "Let's go to the doctor so *she* can fix you." While it may seem harmless at the time, we know that children can internalize these statements as beliefs about who they are and how their health impacts them. The last thing any of us want is for our children to think that something is wrong with them, which causes them to create a mental story about it that defines who they are. We don't want our children to think they're sickly or hyperactive or that there is something wrong with them that only the doctor can fix.

Really pay attention to the language and words you use with your children, because they are listening. Reframe situations for them with positive, affirming statements like:

- "Your body is powerful and knows what it needs. Let's help it help you."
- "You have so much wonderful energy to direct in both fun and useful ways."
- "The doctor helps boost your body's healing powers."

We want to instill trust in our children that their bodies can heal themselves. Whenever things go wrong, as they surely will, then like good detectives, we'll figure out the cause and take action to restore balance.

Now let's discuss three elemental parenting fundamentals: movement, sleep, and screen time. Since healthy eating is such an important topic it is addressed in its own section here and then again in Chapter 5.

Add More Movement

Kids need to be active! They need to be moving at least an hour a day: running around, playing, and having fun. On the one hand, there are the Water and Metal (and sometimes Earth) kids, who enjoy lying about, watching TV, and reading books. On the other hand, there are the Wood, Fire, and (most) Earth kids, who are totally active and on the go all the time. Both sets of kids need to balance activity and rest. Too much activity can make kids overstimulated, overtired, and grumpy, yet the same thing can happen when kids don't get enough activity and have too much screen time.

Since many adults do not get enough exercise, getting your kids moving is a great way to get yourself moving, too! I highly encourage you to create family routines. I take one or both of my boys along with me when I take the dog for walk. It's a great way for me to be mindful and connect with my kids, while also getting exercise for everyone.

It is fairly easy to make sure that kids involved in a sport get enough movement. But there are plenty of ways to get your kids moving even if they aren't interested in team sports. For instance, encourage them to:

- Hop on a pogo stick
- Twirl a hula hoop
- Jump rope
- Have a treasure hunt
- Chase paper airplanes
- Create and run an obstacle course
- Jump on a trampoline
- Have a dance party
- Play a fitness video game like "Dance Party"
- Walk, bike, or scooter to school
- Do yoga or stretching
- Have a water balloon or squirt gun fight
- Toss or kick a ball around

If your kids are open to it, tai chi and qigong are also great ways to incorporate fun and mindful movement in your routine. (You'll find recommendations for books, cards, and websites for both adults and children in the Recommended Resources at the end of this book.) Most important, get out there and move with your kids! They'll be delighted to play with you, and it's a great way to be present with them without distractions.

Limit Screen Time

How much screen time (including computer, TV, video games, and handheld devices) should kids be getting? I think this question is on every parent's mind. We all know when our kids have had too much—they become ornery, irritable, and whiny. It overstimulates their nervous system and can make it hard for any child to settle down and go to bed. In addition, too much screen time can exacerbate any elemental imbalances and affect each element in a different way.

Set clear limits on screen time related to how your particular child responds to watching TV, playing video games, or being online for recreational computer time. For some parents, letting their kids watch TV or play video games only on the weekends is best because their child gets obsessed and it creates upheaval when it's time to turn off the screen. Other kids seem to respond well to having a daily limit.

Wood	Fire	Earth	Metal	Water
Must win, gets super-competitive with others, is obsessed with reaching new level, gets angry when it's time to stop	Gets addicted to the excitement, which exacerbates lack of focus and impulsivity	Thinks obsessively about the game, still thinks about it even after it's turned off	Can't stop thinking about the game, is super-negative and emotional when he loses, can't stop until he gets it perfect	Gets lost in the fantasy world, loses touch with physical needs, forgets to eat and drink, is disconnected from reality

Table 4.1: How Too Much Video Gaming Affects Each Element

Ensure Adequate Sleep

Without a doubt, inadequate sleep can cause kids to be grumpy, irritable, and whiny. However, sleep deprivation in children can often cause surprising symptoms: hyperactivity, impulsivity, and difficulty focusing. Sleep is super important, as it's a time for the body to rest and repair itself and for the brain to form memories and recharge. Children need different amounts of sleep at different ages.

Age	Number of Sleep Hours per Day
0–3 months	14–17
4–11 months	12–15
1–2 years	11–14
3–5 years	10–13
6–13 years	9–11
14–17 years	8–10

Table 4.2: Sleep Duration Recommendations[1]

When your child is getting enough sleep, she'll wake on her own or will easily awaken with an alarm. If you have to repeatedly wake your child, or if she's extremely disoriented and sleepy when you wake her, then she's probably not getting enough sleep. It definitely means your child needs to go to bed earlier, which can mean making adjustments to her overall schedule or creating a ritual to help her fall asleep faster. At least one hour before bed, be sure to dim the lights and avoid screen time.

Having a regular routine for bedtime is very important for all children. Bedtimes shouldn't fluctuate much, even on the weekend. Most routines should include bath, massage, or reading. If possible, keep your child's room dark or allow a dim night-light if needed. Children who have difficulty turning off their thoughts can benefit from quiet activities like reading, coloring, or drawing.

Listening to a guided meditation with progressive relaxation may also be helpful in directing your child's thoughts away from worries or simply quieting her mind. For my recommendations on coloring books, guided meditations, online videos, and other items, visit the Recommended Resources section toward the end of this book.

Each elemental imbalance can present with different issues related to sleep, as shown in Table 4.3. Severe sleep issues are often due to imbalances in multiple elements, and in these cases I recommend seeking the advice of a pediatric acupuncturist.

Wood	Fire	Earth	Metal	Water
Restless sleep, wakes in the middle of the night, or sleeps so deeply she wets the bed	Has trouble falling asleep; can't stop thinking; has restless sleep, light sleep, or vivid dreams	Has obsessive thoughts and worries, can't relax and settle down, needs parents to be with her as she's falling asleep	Has negative thoughts that surface at bedtime, wants to talk about the day when it's time to go to bed, can't relax, can't let go	Can't fall asleep because she's afraid of the dark, afraid of shadows, or has other fears that are worse at night

Table 4.3: How Sleep Issues Manifest According to Elemental Imbalances

Acupressure and Massage

Acupressure and massage are among the easiest things you can do to support your child's health! I highly recommend, no matter what elemental imbalance your child has, doing the nightly Chinese Wellness Massage in Chapter 7. Kids love massage and acupressure, they're easy to do, and they don't require any special tools. They will balance all Five Elements and support the immune system. If your child doesn't have any major imbalances, you can do the wellness massage to keep him healthy and prevent illness.

If he has a specific imbalance, you'll find instructions in Chapter 7 for acupressure points you can massage to correct the imbalances.

I routinely recommend massage and acupressure for the children that I work with in my clinic because both procedures are safe and effective and can be used in addition to Western medical treatments. Plus, they allow bonding time between parent and child that will strengthen the relationship and improve a child's spirit. There's really no downside to daily massage and acupressure.

Special Considerations for Fire and Metal Children

Fire and Metal children are highly sensitive, and this may include sensitivity to touch. Make sure not to touch them so lightly that you tickle them, nor so firmly that the massage is painful. Ask for their feedback during the massage to make sure the pressure you're using is okay, and be sure to explicitly give them permission to tell you if something you're doing is uncomfortable. Massaging these elemental types on a regular basis will help them become less sensitive to touch.

Healthy Eating and Healthy Guts

The health of our children is directly related to the nutrient density of the food they eat. And the food they eat directly affects the health of their gut. A high-quality, nutritious diet will build a strong and healthy body and gut, whereas eating foods high in calories and low in nutrients will lead to imbalances.

In Chapter 5, you'll find in-depth guidance on the foods to avoid and foods to eat for optimal health. You'll also find simple ways you can add nutrition to your child's diet without his even realizing it! However, to get started, these are the highlights:

- Avoid fast foods, white foods, and processed foods
- Avoid artificial colors, flavors, preservatives, and other chemicals
- Eat a rainbow of colors
- Eat with the seasons
- Choose organic foods and organic, free-range meats whenever possible
- Make as much of your food at home as is feasible
- Eat at regular intervals and avoid excessive snacking

Chronic symptoms that don't seem to resolve despite medical care or medication may be related to a food trigger. Food triggers are foods that cause an adverse reaction in the body, resulting in a wide array of symptoms that are unique to each person. They are often the cause of chronic emotional or physical symptoms, such as runny nose, hyperactivity, stomachaches, anxiety, or eczema. Often, simply adding more nutritious foods while removing processed foods, artificial ingredients, and chemical additives can help symptoms resolve. However, if symptoms persist, then it's time to investigate if there's a food trigger. (Chapter 6 goes into more detail on this.)

Any food can cause symptoms, even seemingly healthy foods. In general, children with a Wood imbalance may be more prone to issues with gluten and dairy. Fire and Earth children may have issues with sugar, refined carbohydrates, and food chemicals. Metal children may be more prone to issues with dairy. If your child does have a food trigger, it's also likely negatively impacting his gut flora. When there is an elemental imbalance, food triggers will manifest with a specific set of symptoms, as shown in Table 4.4.

Wood	Fire	Earth	Metal	Water
Headaches, migraines, dizziness, lightheaded-ness, blurry vision, hyperactivity, irritability	Hives, flushing of the face, mood disorders, anxiety, hyperactivity, impulsivity	Digestive problems such as constipation, diarrhea, loose stools, nausea, vomiting, gas, bloating, or fatigue	Dry skin, eczema, runny nose, cough, congestion, frequent illness, asthma, allergies	Being "out of it," depression, low energy, lack of focus, low appetite, stiff or achy joints, dark circles under the eyes

Table 4.4: Food Trigger Symptoms by Element

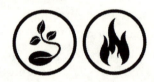

Dietary Considerations for Wood and Fire Kids

Since Wood and Fire children are busy kids, make sure they don't skip meals or grab snacks that offer little nutritional value. Encourage rituals around mealtimes, such as setting the table, to help them relax before eating. These kids need to slow down and chew their food. Fire children especially can eat too quickly, so make sure they're taking time to chew and taste the food they're eating.

Snacks or drinks with sugar or chemicals can quickly create or exacerbate imbalances in the Wood and Fire Elements. These include sodas, sports drinks, energy drinks, processed foods, and sugary foods. Many parents notice their children are hyperactive and irritable after eating too much sugar. This reflects a temporary imbalance in the Wood Element.

Too many fried, rich, and fatty foods are particularly hard on the Wood Element. If your child's Wood Element is deficient, eating berries is very healing. In TCM, we recommend *gou qi zi* berries (also known as goji berries) as a strong tonic for the Wood and Fire Elements. You can find them in most health food stores nowadays.

The Fire child may crave spicy or intensely flavored foods. MSG is a food chemical that intensifies flavors and is very addicting. It is an excitotoxin that can cause behavioral and attention issues, as well as headaches and other physical symptoms. All children should avoid MSG, but if your child has a Fire imbalance, be particularly vigilant about avoiding it.

Dietary Considerations for Earth Kids

Earth children have an affinity for food. Many of them love to cook and immensely enjoy eating, but food can become an issue if your child's Earth Element is out of balance. Make sure that you model healthy eating and portion control. If your child is always hungry, stop and check in with her to find out if she's really hungry or if something else is going on such as upset, boredom, or thirst. Emotional eating may add too many calories to your child's diet and lead to unhealthy weight gain.

If she craves sweets after a meal, make sure she's eating enough protein. If she's hungry after a full meal, it probably means that she's eating too quickly. Encourage her to eat more slowly, smelling and savoring her food. Make her rest 20 to 30 minutes before allowing her to have a second helping. This will allow enough time for her body's "full" signal to reach her brain. If she says she's still hungry after that time, then you'll know it's because she's truly still hungry.

It's a good idea in general not to reward children with food, yet it's something threaded through society. If a child behaves at church, then she gets a doughnut. If she got an A on her paper, we might celebrate with a scoop of ice cream. It seems harmless at the time, but it begins to teach children that food is love. For a child with an Earth imbalance, it's really important to find other ways of rewarding her. Giving your child shared experiences and family connection is a much healthier way of showing her your love.

If your child has an Earth imbalance of any kind, make sure to avoid too many cold, raw foods, and avoid ice-cold drinks. Additionally, make sure she eats at regular intervals. Know that food triggers are extremely common in children with an Earth imbalance.

Dietary Considerations for Metal Kids

Metal children can be extremely picky eaters, with sensitivities to taste and texture. It can definitely try your patience. When a Metal child doesn't like a food, it can seem like he's just being dramatic and making himself gag, but his gag reflex may actually be very forward on the palate. With other children, it may work to force them to sit at the table until they try their peas, but with the Metal child this strategy will backfire. Forcing a Metal child to do anything will result in a battle of wills and turn mealtime into a miserable experience for everyone. I'm not saying you should give in and let him rule dinnertime, but you have to work with him differently. To family members or friends on the outside, it may look like you're giving in to his picky behavior, but in reality, you're helping him develop more flexibility around food.

The strategy I'm going to recommend is what I used to help Noah, my picky eater, overcome his issues with food. It literally took years for him to get used to trying new foods, but now he's much more open to trying new things. Though he adamantly denies liking anything resembling a vegetable, he does eat them now.

Let's say your child refuses to try any green vegetable. He may try to push the broccoli off his plate or get upset when he sees it. At this point, you might think it impossible that he'd willingly try broccoli, and you'd be right. Rather than forcing him to take a bite and risk creating control issues around food, start slowly acclimating your child to the food. Get him simply to be comfortable with having broccoli on his plate without crying. Once he's used to having it on his plate without fussing, then you can have him explore it by first by touching it and eventually smelling it. Then you have him move on to licking it. You may have to stay at each stage for a while before he's ready for the next step. Eventually, have him take a nibble of it and then finally a full bite.

As you go through this process, take the pressure off both yourself and your child by not forcing him to eat the food in question. Make sure there's always something on his plate he enjoys. At least one night each week, make a meal that's super easy and doesn't involve vegetables. Instead, find other ways to work vegetables into his diet. Noah gets a greens supplement with wheat, oat, and barley grasses, which are loaded with vitamins and minerals, as well as fruit and vegetable smoothies. (Just be sure to avoid too many cold, raw foods, especially in the wintertime.) There are also many great cookbooks that have recipes for hiding vegetables in kids' favorite foods; I've listed some of them in the Recommended Resources.

Dietary Considerations for Water Kids

Mealtime is a great way to regularly connect with your Water child. Don't let her tune out during meals by letting her read or watch TV. Instead, use this time to find out what's happening in her daily life at school and in her imaginative inner world.

Support Your Gut Flora, Support Your Health

Increasingly, research is showing how the bacteria in our gut are linked to our immune function, moods, brain function, and nutritional status in addition to digestion. Problems with obesity, asthma, allergies, and mood disorders are now being linked to imbalances in gut flora.[2,3,4,5]

So what are gut flora? They are the bacteria, many of which are beneficial, that live in the gut and have a broad range of functions. Gut flora synthesize vitamins B and K, help digest food, and enable us to absorb minerals like calcium, iron, and magnesium. They feed the cells that make up our gut lining to keep it healthy and strong and prevent pathogens, toxins, and large food particles from getting into our bloodstream and interacting with our immune cells.

Gut flora play a huge role in supporting our immune health. Depending on which source you reference, between 70 and 90 percent of the immune system is in the gut and comes from what's called gut-associated lymphoid tissue (GALT). Gut flora are critical for helping our bodies make important brain chemicals, or neurotransmitters, like dopamine, serotonin, and GABA. Approximately 90 percent of all serotonin is made in the gut, and serotonin is important for mood regulation, sleep, appetite, memory, and learning.[6] The health of our gut flora is critical in creating optimal overall health.

Our gut flora can get out of balance if we:

- Take antibiotics or other medications
- Undergo stress
- Come down with stomach flu or food poisoning
- Have diarrhea or loose stools
- Eat processed foods
- Consume artificial colors, flavors, or sweeteners other chemical additives

Gut flora imbalances will show up differently within each element, as shown in Table 4.5.

Wood	Fire	Earth	Metal	Water
Anger, depression, hyperactivity, impulsivity	Moodiness, mental or emotional disorders, hyperactivity, impulsivity, sleep issues	Abdominal pain, stomachaches, digestive issues, loose stools, constipation, weight gain	Upper respiratory infections or other frequent illness, chronic runny nose or congestion	Lack of emotion, lack of focus, depression, apathy

Table 4.5: Manifestations of Gut Flora Imbalance

If your child has digestive problems, abdominal pain, mental or emotional issues, frequent illness, obesity, asthma, any of the other issues in Table 4.5, or other chronic conditions not mentioned here, then adding probiotics is essential. For children over age two, I recommend a multi-strain daily probiotic with around 25 billion colony forming units (CFU). For children under age two, I recommend a probiotic that is specially formulated for infants. If you're not sure whether probiotics are right for your child, seek the advice of a pediatric acupuncturist or other holistic health-care practitioner. Brands are changing constantly, so please visit www.robinraygreen.com/probiotics for specific recommendations.

Fermented foods such as kefir, homemade yogurt, sauerkraut, kombucha, kimchi, and pickles are another source of probiotics. How many they contain will vary greatly, but consuming them will add variety to your gut flora. Just make sure, if you're buying these products, that they're in the cold section of your store and are not pasteurized. Heat kills good bacteria along with the bad, so pasteurized products won't contain live probiotics.

Natural Remedies

Natural remedies come in many forms; there are herbs, homeo-pathic medicines, and even remedies like lemon socks for fever or poached pears and cinnamon for a dry cough. Often the best natural remedies are preventive in nature or eliminate or reduce our exposure to toxins that cause adverse reactions in the body.

Since all children have unique needs, I won't be discussing specific natural remedies in this book. (However, if you'd like to address a specific complaint your child has, you can visit www .robinraygreen.com and search for the health condition.) All chil-dren, however, can benefit from the natural remedies of acupunc-ture; herbal support; and a healthy, nontoxic home.

Acupuncture and Chinese Herbal Medicine

Acupuncture is an effective way to help your child's body heal and can be used in conjunction with other medical treatments. I've been working with kids for more than a decade, and I can assure you that kids actually do like acupuncture! Contrary to what you might think, it is very easy and painless for children. Pediatric acupuncturists are specially trained in methods devel-oped just for babies and kids, and they use special flexible needles that are as tiny as a strand of hair.

I coined the term *tap* to refer to pediatric needles because of the special technique of rubbing and tapping the acupuncture point before I insert the needle. This desensitizes the point and helps make the experience painless. Also, because most children have negative associations with needles, using that word conjures up images of painful shots or blood draws. Since acupuncture needles are nothing like the hypodermic needles used for shots, using the term *tap* avoids the usual fear and apprehension. "Getting a tap" doesn't seem a bit scary or painful, and once most kids realize this, they're willing to give it a try.

Pediatric acupuncture specialists will take the time to explain what they're doing and help your child understand what is going on. They know how to work with children who may be afraid and can also use techniques that don't involve needles, like low-level cold laser, microcurrent, *tuina*, or *Shonishin*, which stimulate the acupuncture points for a therapeutic effect similar to that of acupuncture.

Most pediatric acupuncturists are trained in Chinese herbal medicine and can prescribe herbal formulas to help speed healing. Like acupuncture, Chinese herbs are very effective for both treating symptoms and resolving the root cause of a health problem. Prescribing an herbal formula starts by first determining the pattern of disharmony and then finding the right herbs that will restore balance and address the health problem. This process is quite specific for each condition and beyond the scope of this book. To find a pediatric acupuncturist in your area, visit www.kidsloveacupuncture.com/directory.

Creating a Healthy, Nontoxic Home

There are thousands of chemicals in the products we buy, and it can be overwhelming to think about all the things we should avoid. I don't expect that we can always avoid all toxins, so I focus on the things that I do have control over: the products I bring into my home, such as household cleaners, detergents, soaps, moisturizers, furniture, mattresses, and food containers. The most important chemicals to know and avoid are phthalates, BPA, formaldehydes, volatile organic compounds (VOCs), and lead. There are simple actions you can take to to reduce your and your family's exposure to these toxins.

1. Make your own household cleaners. Many household cleaners contain toxins such as ammonia, benzenes, chlorine, and formaldehydes. All of these toxins have harmful effects on the body and have been linked to such things as cancer, central nervous system problems, lung damage, and depression.[7] Instead of using store-bought cleaners, make your own at home with natural ingredients such as vinegar, baking soda, and essential oils. There are many free recipes online for effective and safe DIY household cleaners.

2. Avoid plastic food and drink containers. Plastic holds the potential for exposure to phthalates and BPA (bisphenol A), super-toxic chemicals that have been linked to cancer, hormone disruption, neurological damage, and more. Even the BPA replacements in plastics labeled "BPA-free" can also be toxic. In general, try to avoid plastics wherever possible and opt for stainless steel or glass items instead.

3. Limit plastic products for your children in particular. Phthalates are particularly harmful to the brain, hormones, and developing nervous system of a child. They have been associated with ADHD, cancer, thyroid problems, and more. One might assume that because a product is made for babies it's safe, but that's not always the case. In 2009, six types of phthalates were banned for use in children's toys and products; avoid plastic products made before then. If you want to know whether a product contains phthalates or other chemicals, call the manufacturer and check. If you're not sure, don't use the product!

4. Look for low- or no-VOC products to reduce harmful off-gassing. Mattresses, furniture, carpets, paint, and flooring are often sprayed with fire retardants and stain protectors, and these chemicals will release volatile organic compounds (VOCs) in a process known as *off-gassing*. To protect the air quality in your home, purchase items that are labeled low-, no, or zero-VOC. If that's not possible, allow these items to off-gas outside or in a well-ventilated space for several days before bringing them into your home. If you have a baby, wrap her crib mattress in an all-natural wool blanket to prevent the mattress from being a source of toxic exposure for her.

5. Stay clear of potential sources of lead. Lead can be found in some imported toys, painted metal, and toys made in the United States prior to 1978. Avoid very old toys or toys that have been recalled. Any paint in a home built before 1978 is likely to contain lead. Keep children away from peeling or flaking paint, and consider having old paint stripped and redone.

6. Avoid fragrances. The chemicals used in many fragrances, including those in air fresheners, cleaners, and personal care products, are considered VOCs. Many synthetic fragrances can cause allergic reactions, central nervous system disorders, and more.

7. Read labels and ask questions. The most important thing to do is to start reading labels and asking questions about the chemicals in the products we buy. You might be surprised to find known hormone disruptors in your shampoo! Check the label of your personal-care items for these common toxins to avoid:

- Diethanolamine (DEA)
- Triethanolamine (TEA)
- Monoethanolamine (MEA), or ethanolamine
- Nonylphenols
- Parabens (methylparaben, propylparaben, butylparaben)
- Polysorbates
- Polyethylene glycol

Also, check out the website of the Environmental Working Group (www.ewg.org), a nonprofit, nonpartisan organization dedicated to protecting human health and the environment. You'll find wonderful consumer guides of products, foods, toys, and personal care items that are safe for you and your child. For further information on creating a healthy, nontoxic home, please see the Recommended Resources.

Gratitude and Mindfulness

When I first started treating kids, I was surprised to learn that many of them suffer from stress. I guess I thought that kids were somehow invulnerable to stress because they didn't go to work. But the reality is that many kids have intense schedules by the time they reach second grade. They start school early, have structured after-school activities, participate in sports, and do homework. They have little free time to just play and be a kid.

The digital age we live in has brought more stimulation and strong distractions that direct our attention away from being present in the moment. Everywhere we go, adults are checking their e-mail or playing on their phones instead of just being in the moment, and now children are following suit. Many teachers I've spoken with report that in the past couple of decades, children have less-developed social skills and fewer coping skills, which adds to their social and emotional stress at school. Sexual abuse and other traumas, divorce, sibling rivalry, social issues, and trouble at school are great sources of stress for children.

The Wood Element is the first to be affected by stress. Whether it's from hunger, too much homework, a fight with a friend, or family issues, when Wood is affected it can bring about tantrums in babies and younger children and irritability, frustration, headaches, and other physical symptoms in older children. In addition, your child may react with impatience and defiance or become argumentative. Stress can lead to anxiety or sleep problems when it affects Fire; digestive problems and eating issues when it affects Earth; inflexibility and difficulty with change when it affects Metal; and depression, dissociation, and withdrawal when it affects Water.

Coping with stress is an important life skill that will help your child become resilient, and it's something you should model for him every day. We'll always have stress in our lives, but to teach a child how to manage it is probably the most important life skill he can learn. First, teach him to self-regulate both emotionally and physically by balancing activity and rest. It's really important to consider which activities you say yes and no to. Your child will need to find ways to relax. It can be as simple as blowing bubbles, taking a walk, or reading a book. Equally important is teaching relaxation techniques such as breathing, mindfulness, and meditation.

Stress-Proofing with Meditation and Mindfulness

In school, we teach kids to use their logical minds to think, learn, and problem solve. But there's one equally important thing we should be teaching them: how to stop thinking, to quiet their minds, and to just *be*.

Meditation and mindfulness have been around for centuries and are an important aspect of TCM and Eastern philosophies. Mindfulness teaches us to be present in the moment and experience what is happening right now. It helps us become aware of our thoughts and emotions in a nonjudgmental way. Mindfulness can actually reduce anxiety and calm the key area of the brain associated with our stress response, the amygdala, and there's plenty of compelling science to back up its stress-reducing effects.

As life unfolds at a faster and faster pace, it's important for children to have a way to slow down and be present in the moment. Help your children cultivate mindfulness by having them check in with their senses. Ask them: What do you hear right now? What do you smell? What do you feel—a cool breeze or warmth? Take a walk with them and just observe nature. Have them look at the sky, listen to the birds, and feel the air on their skin. Doing this can help them feel more grounded. They'll know they are present in the moment when the voice inside their head stops spinning stories about what they are seeing and instead becomes quiet. As children get older, they often lose this innate ability of being present in the moment, so mindfulness practices can help them keep it.

Teaching your child to meditate is one of the greatest gifts you can give. There are many benefits and compelling science, including MRI brain scans, attesting to the value of this ancient technique. It can help boost the immune system, reduce stress and anxiety, and lower blood pressure.[8, 9, 10] It's helpful for numerous health issues, from digestive problems to skin conditions like psoriasis. But what's really astounding is that meditation can physically change your brain! The more you meditate, the more you increase the gray matter in key areas of the brain related to self-awareness and compassion. Meditation actually helps your brain to become more compassionate and less stressed, even if your external circumstances have not changed a bit!

Experts agree that mindfulness and meditation should be taught to children in school as a way to build emotional intelligence, compassion, and empathy. It can also help children improve their focus and attention, which are the basis for a healthy classroom environment.

When considering meditation, I think most people envision Zen Buddhist meditation, where you sit in the lotus position with the goal of stopping any and all thoughts. However, this is just *one* type of meditation; there are many more that are easy to do and simple to teach. With my boys, I do a simple candle meditation in which I have them focus on a candle flame for a few minutes. For Wood and Fire children, try a walking meditation in which you have them focus on simply breathing and walking. You can also put on a guided meditation designed for children that will help them learn to stop their busy minds and relax. In the Recommended Resources section, I've listed videos, books, and apps with guided meditations that my children enjoy.

The point of these meditations is not to stop your children from thinking, but to direct their focus to something like the candle flame, the guiding voice, the breathing and walking. Their minds will still have thoughts, but as they notice them, they simply redirect their minds back to the object of focus. This is what helps reduce stress and improve focus. In the beginning, this can be really hard, but reassure your kids that, just like building any skill, the more they practice, the easier it becomes.

Meditation and mindfulness are powerful forms of medicine. As public awareness of the benefits grows, I believe meditation will become a regular, daily habit that we instill in our children just like brushing their teeth, eating healthful foods, and getting enough sleep.

Fostering Grateful Children

Gratitude is the basis of happiness. This practice allows us to appreciate the journey rather than only looking forward to the destination. Modern society leans toward always striving for the next thing that will make us happy. It leads us to believe that something outside of ourselves will fulfill us. For kids, it may be when they get that shiny red bike, that cool outfit, or the latest and greatest video game. The truth is that these things provide temporary gratification but will leave us and our children feeling empty and wanting more.

Gratitude teaches us that regardless of our external circumstances or challenges, we have things in our lives that are of value right now. It teaches us to be happy no matter what. Much of our suffering comes from the judgments we make about what we do or don't have. Developing our gratitude muscle helps avert this type of suffering by teaching us to find the positive in our lives right now.

We can have gratitude for all the simple pleasures in life and see that every moment we have is a gift. When we're distracted by thoughts of the past or wants for the future, we miss out on the beauty that is in front of us right now. Gratitude can ground us in the present and help us see all the many blessings we have.

The best way to teach gratitude is to model it for our children and express our gratitude for the blessings in our lives. It can be for the amazing things that happen to us, or it can be for the simple pleasures of being alive. We can express gratitude for a summer breeze, a beautiful sunset, or the crickets chirping. We can express gratitude for our food and water, perhaps by saying a simple blessing.

I recommend fostering the habit of gratitude by adopting one or more of these simple practices recommended by gratitude researcher and author Christine Carter, Ph.D.:

- At dinner go around the table and have everyone share something for which they're grateful.
- Ask your child to tell you about "three good things" that happened that day (bedtime is a great time for this).
- Create a "gratitude box." Have your child write down something she is grateful for on a slip of paper and put it in the box every day. Read all the "gratitude fortunes" once a week.[11]

Gratitude doesn't have to be a formal practice; it can be simply a way of being in the world. Passing on this quality to your children will help them live a full and blessed life in which they can enjoy the journey and all the stops along the way. All parents want their children to be happy and healthy, and developing a daily habit of gratitude is a surefire way to see that they are.

Provide Preventive Seasonal Support

Each element corresponds with a particular season. If an element is out of balance, it will likely get worse during the corresponding season. You may also notice improvements or challenges in your child's health according to the season of her Dominant Element. For example, if you have a Metal child, you may notice that she has more dry skin and head colds in the fall; if you have a

Fire child, you may see an increase in her impulsive nature during the summertime.

Wood	Fire	Earth	Metal	Water
Spring	Summer	Late summer* or end of each season	Fall	Winter

Table 4.6: Most Challenging Seasons for Each Element

*Late summer refers to the end of summer and beginning of fall, the time of harvest and celebration.

Imbalances that worsen with the corresponding season can help point you toward what you need to do to support your child during that time. The Wood child will need to get plenty of physical activity, eat lots of healthy foods, and avoid food chemicals in the spring. The Fire child needs support in the form of physical activity, meditation, and mindfulness to help her overcome her impulsive tendencies in the summer. The Earth child needs extra digestive support at the change of the seasons and in late summer. The Metal child needs extra immune support, probiotics, and a healthy diet going into fall. And the Water child will need to stay active in the winter or risk becoming depressed.

By noticing the seasonal patterns related to the health challenges they face, we can be proactive in helping our kids improve their health. Then, we can take measures to support our child to have a smooth season. In Chapter 5, you'll find specific dietary recommendations to support your child's element, and you can use the acupressure points and massage techniques outlined in Chapter 7 to support your child's element during their challenging season.

Putting It All Together

If this feels like a lot of information, you may be thinking, *How the heck am I going to do all those things you just recommended to heal my whole child? Where do I even start?*

I always tell the parents I'm working with to start with the easiest practices. Would adding a massage routine at bedtime be easy and help your child with her sleep issues? Would switching out just a few items in your child's diet eliminate many of the artificial ingredients in it? Do those things first.

Now it's time to create a longer-term plan to help restore elemental balance and harmony in your child. In order to do that, you need to fill in the healing program template in Appendix C. For an example, you can go to Appendix D to see the plan I used to treat Noah's eczema. You can also download the questionnaires and template at www.robinraygreen.com/healyourchild. For more background information and to create a full treatment plan, be sure to continue reading.

CHAPTER FIVE

Build a Foundation for Optimal Health

Mealtime is one way we can make a significant impact on the direction of our children's health. Make sure to carve out time in your weekly schedule to sit down and dine with your children. It is a wonderful opportunity to gather and bond with your family. Conversation not only helps us bond emotionally but also slows us down as we eat, giving our stomachs time to tell our brains that we're full. Mealtime is when we have the most control over our children's diet, and we can provide foods that are easy to digest, are rich in nutrients, and support healthy gut flora and immunity.[1]

We literally are what we eat. As one health practitioner and friend says, "Garbage in, garbage out." If we eat foods that are extensively processed, full of chemicals, and devoid of nutrients, we'll feel just like the food we're eating: tired, sick, and full of garbage. Processed foods containing additives, preservatives, and chemical ingredients actually rob the body of nutrients. They impact the gut, which we know from Chapter 4 is essential to having a healthy, well-functioning immune system.

Nutrients from our children's diet are the building blocks for their bones, skin, muscles, brain tissue, organs, and glands. Children who eat nutrient-rich diets have fewer allergies, behavioral issues, mood disorders, chronic illness, depression, fatigue, and digestive troubles. It's also important that children eat at regular intervals so their blood sugar level remains stable. Going too long between meals or constantly snacking can lead to issues with blood sugar or weight.

Food is medicine. It heals, it cures, and it prevents illness. A good diet enables the Earth Element to break down, transform, and transport nutrients to nourish each and every cell in the body. Good food supports the Water Element to ensure proper growth and development. When the Earth and Water Elements are healthy and balanced, the Metal Element is nourished, leading to a healthy immune system and resilience to infectious disease and illness.

Forsaking Nutrition for Convenience

Starting in the 1950s, processed foods—foods that were altered, precooked, and prepackaged for convenience—began gaining ground in the American diet. By the 1970s, the sale and consumption of processed foods had exploded. Increasingly, families had both parents entering the workforce, and it was liberating to be able to buy inexpensive and easy-to-prepare food. Microwave ovens became cheaper and more popular, and even kids could "nuke" frozen meals quickly and easily.

At the time, we didn't know how bad these foods were or were going to get. We didn't realize that we were becoming addicted to all the salt, fat, and sugar, and giving up our health for the sake of convenience. As processed foods seep into every corner of the grocery store, chronic illnesses and inflammatory diseases that once mainly affected adults have begun to impact our children as well.

Around the same time processed food was becoming a household staple, we had a cultural shift regarding medicine. We started to believe that we could use a drug to treat any symptom and cure any illness. We didn't realize that we were causing many of those symptoms and illnesses ourselves with poor diet, sedentary lifestyle, and lack of self-care. Our grandparents and their grandparents, on the other hand, had believed strongly in the power of food as medicine. Before antibiotics, vaccines, and pharmaceuticals, generations relied on food to cure simple illness and speed up healing.

Traditional homemade foods are usually rich in nutrients that support healing, reduce inflammation, and increase our resilience to illness. In cultures all over the world, you'll find dishes like bone broths, soaked and sprouted nuts and grains, and other foods that take extra time and care to prepare. Remedies like honey and lemon to soothe a sore throat and calm a cough, and spicy foods to make us sweat and treat a head cold, were often abandoned as we became more reliant on modern medicine.

I'm happy to report that we are coming full circle now, realizing how important healthy eating is to preventing illness in the first place. But we have to work harder to get access to the healing foods we need. The grocery store is a completely different world from what it was 50 years ago, and parents have to be expert label readers in order to ensure they're choosing healthy foods. Deceitful labeling makes it hard to tell what is good for you and what's not, but once you know what to look for, it gets easier to pick healthy items.

The Consequences of the Processed-Food Diet

Being "overfed and malnourished" is an increasingly common condition nowadays that's associated with obesity and other health problems. Quite simply, it means that even though a person may be consuming enough calories (or more than enough), the poor quality of the food she's eating may be leading to conditions such as nutrient deficiencies, inflammation, diabetes, and general unwellness. Many of us overconsume processed, prepackaged foods that are high in sugar, salt, and fat and packed with additives, preservatives, and other chemicals to enhance taste and texture and prolong shelf life. Eating this way negatively impacts the gut, immune system, and resistance to disease.

The statistical evidence is staggering. Children born today have a much higher chance of developing a chronic illness or mood disorder in childhood than their parents did. One third of all kids in the United States are diagnosed with ADHD, allergies, asthma, or autism. Almost one-fifth will be diagnosed with a serious mental disorder such as depression.[2] Assuming their diet and environment remain constant, nearly half of children born in this century will become obese or overweight, and one in three will eventually suffer from diabetes.[3] This doesn't even include other diseases related to poor diet, including mood and behavioral disorders, recurrent pain, autoimmune diseases, digestive disorders, tooth decay, and cancer. Nutrient deficiencies and exposure to toxins, even when not the root cause of these problems, only make these conditions worse.

There is one huge thing that we can do today to start alleviating the problem: change what we're feeding our kids.

The Pillars of a Good Diet

A good diet is based on real foods that are easy to digest and support healthy gut flora. It contains foods that are anti-inflammatory and rich in vitamins, minerals, antioxidants, and probiotics. It minimizes our exposure to chemical ingredients and pesticides, thereby reducing our body's toxic load, and it includes clean or purified water.

These pillars of a good diet are based on the work of researcher Weston A. Price. (For a more thorough discussion of these pillars, see "Principles of Healthy Diets" at the Weston A. Price Foundation website: www.westonaprice.org.) In the 1920s, Dr. Price noticed an alarming pattern of dental irregularities, including cavities, crooked teeth, and bite issues. He suspected that these "dental deformities," as he called them, were due to either genetics or poor nutrition from the modern diet. To test his theory, he studied the varied diets of preindustrialized peoples who didn't have dental deformities and didn't suffer from common Western degenerative diseases such as cancer, heart disease, or diabetes.

What Dr. Price found was that when processed foods entered the food supply of these people, they immediately showed signs of physical degeneration similar to those seen in Western industrialized cultures. Dr. Price documented his findings with more than 15,000 photos, taken over two to three generations, that depict a shift in tooth and facial structure and an increase in Western diseases as modern foods were increasingly eaten.[4]

To simplify Dr. Price's pillars of a good diet, we can look to the work of Katherine Erlich, M.D., and Kelly Genzlinger. In their book, *Super Nutrition for Babies*, Erlich and Genzlinger advise us that the food we eat must ultimately be:

- Digestible
- Pure
- Immune boosting
- Nutrient dense[5]

How do we teach our children to decipher the challenging world of food? I have found that using the concept of red, yellow, and green lights is very effective and fun.

Red-, Yellow-, and Green-Light Foods

The red-, yellow-, and green-light system is simple for kids to understand and easy to use in categorizing foods. It can help your children make healthy choices when you're not around to guide them. While it is similar in name to the "traffic light diet" used by Leonard H. Epstein and his colleagues to manage childhood obesity, the focus in this book is not weight loss, but rather helping kids easily identify foods that fit within the pillars of a good diet and provide optimal nutrition. I frequently use the red/yellow/green analogy in my own clinic.

- *Red-light foods* should rarely be eaten. You might save these for special occasions like birthdays, or as a rare treat.
- *Yellow-light foods* should be eaten with caution. You can eat them occasionally, but don't make them a regular part of your grocery list.
- *Green-light foods* can be eaten as often as you want. You get a free pass!

What happens to children when they eat the standard American diet, composed primarily of red- and yellow-light foods? Well, I think we're clearly seeing the consequences now: obesity, diabetes, chronic inflammatory diseases, frequent illness, tooth decay, behavioral and mood issues, and pediatric cancer, to name just a few. Not only does this diet fail to provide proper nutrition and contribute to the toxic burden children carry; it also actually blocks nutrients from being absorbed—the very nutrients babies and children need for proper growth, development, and immune function. They contribute to the state of being "overfed and malnourished." If something doesn't change, the social cost will be enormous. But there is hope, and it comes in the form of green-light foods.

Green-Light Foods

Green-light foods are the ideal foods we should have in our diets. They are often referred to as "real foods" and "whole foods." Real foods are pure and haven't been altered or sprayed with chemicals. They don't contain preservatives, so they tend to have a short shelf life. They're also nutrient dense and especially good for promoting healing and supporting immunity. They are free of toxins and packed with a wide array of antioxidants, vitamins, and minerals. They supply inflammation fighters and are often a source of fat-soluble mineral activators that allow the body to absorb and use minerals. Many also contain probiotics and enzymes to promote digestibility.[6]

Green-light foods support proper brain growth and aid in cognitive and immune system development. They have protective and regenerating effects on the body and can actually restore health![7] I encourage every parent I work with to include more of these foods in their child's diet, especially when the child is recovering from an acute or chronic illness. When a child is eating mostly green-light foods, the yellow light foods they eat don't have much of an effect on their health because they're still getting enough nutrients.

Grains, Legumes, Nuts, and Seeds	Whole, sprouted, soaked, or leavened varieties
Fruits and Vegetables	Organic and local varieties
Fats	Unrefined and cold-pressed olive oil or avocado oil or tropical fats like coconut and palm
Dairy	100% whole-fat milk, whole milk yogurt, and homemade dairy products made from organic, grass-fed, and raw or low-temperature-pasteurized milk
Meat	Pasture-raised and/or grass-fed beef, pork, and poultry; eggs from these hens; and gelatin made from pasture-raised, grass-fed animals
Seafood	Wild-caught fish, shellfish, clams, oysters, mussels, scallops, anchovies, and sardines
Traditional Superfoods	Liver and other organ meats from pastured, organically raised animals; cod liver oil; bone marrow and mineral-rich bone broths; fish roe (fish eggs)
Fermented Foods	Probiotic-rich condiments such as chutney, sauerkraut, and pickles
Beverages	Lacto-fermented ginger ale, kefir drinks, and kombucha
Soy	Fermented soy sauce, tempeh, miso

Table 5.1: Green-Light Foods

An easy way to find green-light foods is to shop the perimeter of the grocery store, as this is generally where all the real, whole foods are located: the produce section, meat and dairy cases, and bulk bins of nuts, grains, etc. The interior aisles generally have the processed and junk foods, because they're loaded with preservatives to be shelf-stable. Be sure to read all the labels on any packaged and prepared products you buy. Also, make more foods at home, so you can know what ingredients are used and control the quality.

Choose bread made from ancient grains such as kamut, spelt, or einkorn that is properly leavened or fermented. Look for breads with labels that indicate they're made in small batches using the old fashioned sourdough or leavening processes. You'll find this bread higher in nutrients and easier to digest.

I also recommend eating mostly soaked and sprouted nuts, which are sometimes called "activated" nuts. In order for us to get nourishment from nuts, they must be soaked for about eight hours and then rinsed to remove the phytic acid from their protective covering. This covering prevents them from sprouting but also makes them difficult to digest and blocks nutrients from being absorbed. There are many simple recipes for soaking and sprouting your own nuts.

When it comes to fruits and vegetables, be sure to ask where these items have come from, and shop at your local farmers' market as much as possible. Know what's in season; if you find produce that's out of season, it may have been shipped in from another country.

When milk is sourced from clean and humane dairy farms where the cows are free to roam the pasture and eat their native diet of grass, milk is everything it's promised to be. Raw, whole milk really does do a body good, because it's loaded with vitamins, minerals, protein, and enzymes and has immune-boosting factors that make it a nutritional powerhouse. If you live in an area where raw milk is not available, opt for low-temperature pasteurization where possible.

When purchasing meat, ask the butcher where the meat comes from and whether the animal was raised in a pasture and grass fed. Does the label say organic or, if you're in the United States, USDA organic?

Bone broth and gelatin contain collagen, which helps nail, hair, and skin growth. Drinking homemade bone or vegetable broth and eating gelatin are really easy ways to help heal the gut with food.

Cultured, or fermented, foods support digestive health because they add good bacteria to the gut. Cultured foods include sauerkraut, fermented fruits and vegetables, fermented dairy like kefir and yogurt, and fermented beverages like kombucha and kefir soda. When buying cultured or fermented foods, especially vegetables, buy the kind that are unpasteurized and located in the refrigerated section of the grocery store. If pickles or sauerkraut have been pasteurized, they've been heated, which kills both bad and beneficial bacteria.

When buying soy products, be sure to choose those that are fermented, like tempeh, because soy products that are not fermented have a high phytic-acid content.

Yellow-Light Foods

Yellow-light foods are in the middle of the spectrum. They can be eaten sometimes, but not all the time, because they're not as pure, whole, digestible, or nutrient dense as their green-light counterparts. Yellow-light foods are everywhere from the grocery store to the restaurant on the corner because they're cheap and convenient. Yellow-light foods aren't inherently bad for you, but their quality has been compromised, often to increase production. For instance, conventionally grown fruits and vegetables, while nutritious, come with a higher chemical load from pesticide residues than their organic counterparts.[8] Chemicals might also be used on or in the food to preserve shelf life or enhance taste or texture. And yellow-light foods are typically not prepared in a way that makes them easy to digest. For example, the roasted nuts from the grocery store haven't been soaked and sprouted to increase their nutrition and make them easier for our bodies to process.[9]

It's fine to have some yellow-light foods in your children's diet, but be sure that these foods don't make up your entire shopping list.

Grains, Legumes, Nuts, and Seeds	Whole but unsoaked, unsprouted, or unleavened varieties
Fruits and Vegetables	Conventionally or internationally grown varieties
Fats	Refined and nonorganic cold-pressed olive oil or tropical fats like coconut and palm
Dairy	Nonorganic 100% whole-fat milk, whole milk yogurt, and premade dairy products made from cows raised without hormones or antibiotics
Meat	Organic, corn-fed beef, pork, and poultry; and eggs from these hens
Seafood	Farmed fish, shellfish, clams, oysters, mussels, scallops, and sardines
Preserved Foods	Dried fruits and meat jerky with preservatives
Fermented Foods	Pasteurized pickles, sauerkraut, kimchi

Table 5.2: Yellow-Light Foods

One big thing to conquer when it comes to yellow-light foods is whole grain bread. There is so much advertising touting whole grains as super-duper healthy for us, yet most whole grain products aren't properly prepared and still have a high glycemic index, meaning they spike blood sugar levels because the body rapidly breaks them down into glucose. Nuts and grains that haven't been soaked, sprouted, soured, or leavened in a way that removes phytic acid are definitely yellow-light foods because you can't access their full nutrition.

Nonorganic vegetables and fruits contain pesticide residues, sometimes from 13 or more chemicals.

When it comes to dairy products, the pasteurization process destroys enzymes and vitamins that would make them more nutritious, which is why companies have to add nutrients back into the milk. Pasteurized dairy products are also more irritating to the digestive tract. Organic, whole-fat dairy products are better than low-fat and nonfat products.

Organic meats are better than traditional because the animals are not fed antibiotics and can eat their natural diet. Conventional eggs come from factory farms where the hens are kept in confined spaces under inhumane living conditions, fed a corn feed, and often given antibiotics. (Know, however, that even if eggs are labeled "free range," it doesn't guarantee a higher standard of living conditions for the hens; it's always best if you can ask the farmer yourself.) Farmed fish live in unnaturally confined spaces as well, which is why they are often dosed with antibiotics; wild-caught is preferred.

Soy products generally have a high phytic-acid content, which is why I recommend fermented soy products only. Diets with an excess of unfermented soy products can cause dangerous zinc and iron deficiencies that have long-term adverse effects in children.

One big step when it comes to discovering yellow-light foods is acknowledging that many food products have deceptive labels. You'll find "Contains Whole Grains" proudly stamped on the front of a label, yet when you turn the package over, you learn that enriched wheat flour is the main ingredient. A product can be mostly refined white flour, but as long as the food manufacturer adds a certain percentage of whole wheat flour, it can be called a whole grain product.

Before starting my journey, I never carefully looked at the label on the bread I was buying. When I finally did, I found a lot of ingredients I didn't recognize, including additives and preservatives to go along with those whole grains. Some holistic health and medical experts refer to the push for Americans to eat whole grains as the "whole grain hoax."

What happened to our bread? By the 1960s, most commercial bakeries had done away with the process of using yeast to ferment the grains in a slow-rise fashion that made the grains more digestible.[10, 11] Instead, commercial bakeries began using a high-pressure aeration process with chemical additives that allowed them to make a loaf of bread in under three hours. Also, changes had been made in the wheat plant through hybridization in order to increase crop yield. According to the Broadbalk Wheat Experiment, which tracked the nutritional content of wheat since 1843, current wheat has a lower nutritional profile than the wheat we ate prior to the 1960s. Similar to raw milk, wheat in its original form is everything it's promised to be, but in its processed form it's a cheap knockoff.

Red-Light Foods

Red-light foods typically are high in fat, salt, and sugar and come out of a package. Chemicals are added to the red-light foods to extend the shelf life and create a pleasing texture. They're red light because we want our kids to STOP before they put it in their mouths!

Some red-light foods may surprise you, like nonorganic, low-fat, pasteurized dairy, and sugar-laden low-fat yogurts. Doesn't dairy do a body good? Don't kids need it to build strong bones? The problem is that pasteurized milk can irritate the digestive tract and promote inflammation. High-temperature pasteurization not only kills harmful bacteria in milk that is created from industrial dairy farms but also destroys the enzymes that help us digest milk and depletes the very nutrients that make it so healthy.

Cereals are all red-light. Regardless of whether they are touted as healthy or organic, like products made by Kashi or Cascadian Farms, all cereals are highly processed and heated to high temperatures. Vitamins must be added back in by the manufacturers. Even cereals thought of as healthy may contain genetically modified soy, as in soy protein isolate or natural flavorings.

Grains	White breads, crackers, cereal, bagels; anything made with bleached, refined white flour
Sweeteners	High-fructose corn syrup, sucrose, sugar, artificial sweeteners such as saccharine, aspartame, and sucralose
Snacks	Cereal bars, protein bars, granola bars
Fats	GMO oils or imitation butters; soy, corn, canola, and cottonseed oils; margarine and butter substitutes
Dairy	Nonorganic, pasteurized low-fat and nonfat milk and yogurt; premade dairy products made from cows raised with hormones and antibiotics
Meat	Nonorganic beef, pork, and poultry and deli meats; eggs from factory-farmed hens
Salt	Refined white salt
Beverages	Sodas; store-bought juices; drinks laden with sugar, high-fructose corn syrup, or artificial sweeteners like flavored waters and sports drinks
Soy	Unfermented products such as soy milk, soy snacks, and soy protein

Table 5.3: Red-Light Foods

Striving for Balance: Adding More Green While Reducing Red

In Appendix D you'll find a list of simple switches that can help your family go from red-light to green-light foods without too much fuss. Make consistent incremental changes, and most important, take back your food and your kitchen and make every bite count! Eating real, nutrient-dense foods is the key to reversing illness and helping kids grow healthy bodies.

The reality is, however, that we'll probably never completely rid our diet of red-light foods. We live in the modern world, and no matter where we go, red-light foods are there. Sometimes we're faced with a bad food choice or a *worse* food choice, so we just do the best we can with what we have at the moment. Ideally, we should strive for 80 percent green-light foods, 20 percent yellow- and red-light foods. But we may start out at 60:40 or 70:30, and that's fine. We can continually make changes to get to a better ratio.

Remember, we teach by example. If your spouse or teenagers are super resistant to changing their diet, it can sabotage your efforts. If that's the case, then it's time to sit down and have a talk about why you're making changes, how the new diet will help their bodies, and the example they are setting for your children (or, in the case of teenagers, their younger siblings). Your spouse is an adult, so he or she can eat red-light foods outside the house, but you should agree on which foods don't come inside.

Sometimes red-light foods can be the vehicle for green-light foods, as when conventional store-bought corn chips are eaten with guacamole made at home with fresh organic produce. But there are often healthier, more nutritious versions of red-light foods that we can reach for, and we can make over our favorite processed-food meals to become healthier green-light versions. If pizza is a favorite, you can start by making your own leavened pizza dough and homemade sauce and adding raw organic cheese. Instead of eating out, make hamburgers at home with buns fresh from your local bakery. We turned Taco Tuesday at our house into a completely green-light meal. We make our own refried beans, guacamole, salsa, and cashew cheese sauce. We use organic tortilla chips and grass-fed, organic ground beef with our own blend of spices. It definitely takes more planning and work, but it is totally worth it. Taco Tuesday has never been more delicious and healthy!

There's also nothing wrong with choosing to spend your time with your family instead of in the kitchen! Most of us no longer make our own bread, tortillas, or crackers from scratch. We just need to become expert label readers so that we can make better choices.

I feel that eating healthy is not only a journey but an awakening. First, you realize you're not eating as well as you thought. You start turning the box or jar around and read what's actually in the foods you're buying. You're aghast when you find out that what you thought was healthy is actually *crap*. Then you get angry. Really pissed off! How dare the food companies lie to me! Isn't the FDA supposed to be watching our backs? Isn't there a law against deceitful labeling? How can this soda be labeled "all natural" when there's not a single natural ingredient in it?

Then you mourn your old way of eating, until finally you reach acceptance. You accept that nobody is looking out for your family's diet but *you*. We can blame the food companies all we want, but we're the ones buying the processed foods. When you reach acceptance, you start on the journey of cleaning up your diet and clearing out the foods you once thought were healthy. You take back control of your family's diet, and it feels awesome! At first it won't be easy—and not everyone may be on board—but slowly things will turn around, and you'll be a healthier, happier family.

The first step to reducing the red-light foods in your family's diet is to read labels and recognize where they're hiding. In the beginning, this switch can be time-consuming and exasperating. However, the more you do it, the better you'll get at it, the wiser you'll be to the tricks of food marketers, and the less you'll be prey to the gimmicks they use.

The second step is to make simple switches that your family won't really notice. For instance, identify the food items that you're buying out of habit that can easily be made at home, often for a fraction of the cost. My family started making seasoning mixes and salad dressings from organic ingredients rather than purchasing premade versions, which contain MSG, GMOs, and artificial colors and flavors. You can switch from quick-cooking oatmeal to soaking whole oats overnight to unlock their nutrients. Continue to make small, consistent changes to your family's diet, and before you know it, they'll be eating healthier without even realizing it. Then, as you reach a new level of healthy eating, you'll become aware of additional switches that you can make and you'll go even healthier.

The third step is to change the way you shop and cook. We need to make meal preparation an event that engages the whole family. You'll quickly get used to the planning and prep that go into making meals from scratch. Cooking and cleaning together can actually be a wonderful time to connect with your kids, giving them lifelong skills that will continually serve them. You don't want your child going off to college having no idea how to cook an egg or make a basic meal. The more you do it, the faster and easier it becomes.

Having the kids involved in making food has been a delight for me and my husband. Even though Noah is not wild about vegetables, ever since he's been cooking with us, he's been so much more open to at least trying new foods. And every now and then, he finds a new food that he really likes and that broadens his diet just a little bit more.

If you and your partner both work, you may be thinking that you don't have time to prepare healthy meals. But cooking healthy isn't about slaving away in the kitchen all day; it's about planning, preparing, and cooking smarter so you work less and enjoy your food and your family more. You'll need to adopt a new weekly pattern and create time in your schedule to do the prep work so you can quickly make healthy meals during the busy week. Whether you work or not, planning and preparing on the weekends will make a huge difference in making healthy meals happen. Here are a few tips to get you started on your real-food journey:

— *Weekend planning and preparation:* It's important to use part of the weekend (or whatever days you have off) to plan your meals, shop for ingredients, and do all the prep you can to make it easier during the week to throw a meal together. Prepare any ingredients that may take hours or days. For instance, our refried beans take at least a full day in the slow cooker before they're ready.

— *Batch cooking:* Batch cooking means you take several hours on one day to prepare meals for the next few days, so all you have to do is reheat and eat. Doing this has saved our bacon, so to speak, many times.

— *Slow-cooker meals:* Nothing beats coming home to a meal that's been simmering all day in the slow cooker. I recommend getting a cookbook with healthy slow-cooker meal ideas. It can make your life so much easier.

— *Dressed-up leftovers:* Transform your leftovers into a new meal. Make two to three extra-large dishes a week, and repurpose leftovers. For instance, cook a whole chicken and have that one night with a salad or veggies, then shred the rest of the meat and use it another night in a taco salad, wraps, burritos, or a soup.

— *Meal planning subscriptions:* Sometimes we lack inspiration or don't have the time to create meal plans with ideas for leftovers. Not to worry! There are many healthy meal plan subscriptions you can purchase that will save you the work of figuring out what's for dinner (see Recommended Resources for websites). Most of these come with a weekly meal plan, shopping lists, and ideas for making leftover meals. Most are scalable to you family's special dietary needs, size, and budget.

All of these things will take a little more effort, but you'll gradually shift your family's diet over to more green-light foods. My patients are always relieved to find out that it took me a couple of years to completely revamp my family's diet. It wasn't as if it happened in a day, a week, or even a month. It took time. Give yourself permission to take your time on this journey.

When I began my real-food journey, I went through all the stages I mentioned above. In the end, knowing is so much better than not knowing. If you've been feeding your family mostly red-light foods, don't beat yourself up. You didn't know what you didn't know. But now you can start making changes that will have a positive effect on your health and the health of your kids. Even if at first they're not wild about the new food paradigm, they'll eventually come around.

Three Dietary Changes That Have the Biggest Impact

Information on what to avoid and why you should avoid it could fill an entire book, and it is certainly way more than I can cover in this chapter without overwhelming you! I don't want you to feel as if you're so far removed from eating healthy that you give up before you've started. Start with incremental changes that are easy to make. I've narrowed it down to the top three things you can change to have the greatest impact.

For more information on food chemicals, tricky labeling, and easy switches to improve the quality and nutrient density of common foods that kids love to eat, visit www.robinraygreen.com.

Change 1: Avoid Chemicals in Your Food

When it comes to avoiding chemicals in your food, Michael Pollan, a real-food advocate, says it best: "Avoid food products containing ingredients that a third-grader cannot pronounce." Can you say monoammonium glutamate (yet another sneaky name for MSG), transglutaminase (also called "meat glue"), tertiary butylhydroquinone (TBHQ), or butylated hydroxytoluene (BHT)? Seriously, what the heck are these chemicals doing in our food? Once you start reading labels, you'll find all kinds of interesting names that are unpronounceable and certainly not recognizable. If they're not ingredients you'd keep in the pantry, a good rule of thumb is to avoid them in the food you buy.

Most prepackaged foods and virtually all fast foods contain chemicals, including preservatives, additives, texture enhancers, artificial colors, and artificial flavorings. Most food companies justify the use of these ingredients by saying they're not used in large enough amounts to negatively impact our health. But if you're eating foods with these ingredients in a few meals each day, your exposure adds up. No one really knows exactly what a combination of these additives will do to a child's body, which is more sensitive to chemicals than the adult body is. When it comes to food dyes, the FDA states that there isn't conclusive evidence linking artificial food dyes to ADHD, but the European Union requires food containing artificial dyes to be labeled "May have an adverse effect on activity and attention in children."[12]

It's difficult to know whom and what to trust. American food companies will assert that certain food additives are safe for the general public, even though these same chemicals (e.g., BHT and TBHQ) have been banned in Europe, Australia, and Japan. Various additives have been linked to digestive problems, skin problems, asthma, allergic reactions, hyperactivity, and cancer. Even when companies in other countries have found safer alternatives, the harmful additives are still used in American foods.

One time, my son Nate drank blue Gatorade, and within 20 minutes he was vibrating and couldn't sit still! I'd never seen him act like that before, and we realized that it was probably the blue food dye. Since that incident, we make sure to steer clear of fake colors in our food and drink. The most important thing we can do is to trust our parental instincts on how our children will react to certain foods, regardless of what is said to be safe.

It's our job to look out for our children's health and avoid as many of these ingredients as possible. Watch out for:

- *Preservatives:* TBHQ, EDTA, BHA, BHT, nitrates, nitrites, sulfites, sulfates
- *Flavor Enhancers:* natural and artificial flavors, MSG
- *Texture Enhancers:* carrageenan, L-cysteine
- *Enhanced Food Appeal:* artificial food dyes

Fast foods are a hotbed of chemical additives. From the bun to the beef to the fries, a fast-food meal is a veritable chemical concoction. I would recommend avoiding any and all fast food for that reason alone. For more complete information on food chemicals to avoid, see Appendix E.

Change 2: Eat Locally Grown and
Organic Foods When Possible

Some experts claim that organic foods are no different from conventionally grown food. I certainly wouldn't want to waste my grocery budget on more expensive food if it's not any better or safer! The problem is that there's nothing conventional about "conventionally" grown foods. Most of these come from farms that use pesticides on their crops. In many cases, they don't use just one pesticide. According to the Environmental Working Group, certain foods like cherry tomatoes, peaches, and nectarines were found to have 13 different pesticide residues! And now that our grocery stores have gone global, there's no way for us to know with certainty what pesticides have been sprayed on the foods we're eating, especially those coming from countries with less strict laws governing pesticide usage.

I live near Watsonville, California, which is known for growing strawberries, one of the most pesticide-laden fruits in the produce section. The farm workers have to wear protective gear that looks like a space suit in order to spray a class of pesticides called fumigants. Inhaling these toxic fumes is linked to cancer, respiratory damage, neurotoxicity, and more. This horrifies me because strawberries are a kid favorite. Can you imagine your child eating a strawberry after it's been sprayed? What level of poison is safe for your child? In my opinion, those who argue against organic foods have missed the point. There is no level of pesticide that feels safe for me to allow my kids to eat.

The American Academy of Pediatrics confirms that children are especially vulnerable to the toxicity of pesticides, and states, "Prenatal and early childhood exposure to pesticides is associated with pediatric cancers, decreased cognitive function and behavioral problems." Research studies on organophosphates from pesticides show that chronic, low-level exposure may affect neurodevelopment and growth in children. According to a 2012 study published in the *Annals of Allergy, Asthma and Immunology,* higher levels of exposure to dichlorophenols, chlorine compounds used in pesticides and chlorinated water, may contribute to increasing rates of food allergies in industrialized nations.[13] Organic fruits and vegetables aren't trendy or just a marketing ploy—they are absolutely necessary for the health of our children!

Organic foods are the real traditional foods. Ideally, they are grown in a sustainable way that doesn't harm our environment, enriches the land, and leads to healthy plants that can resist disease without toxic chemical protection. When you buy organic produce, it's not just about the nutritional content but about avoiding the worst toxins. According to the USDA website, "Synthetic fertilizers, sewage sludge, irradiation, and genetic engineering may not be used" on products calling themselves organic. Unfortunately, organic farming doesn't mean that foods are chemical-free or pesticide-free, because they are still allowed to use organic pesticides. But overall, organic foods contain less pesticides than their conventionally grown counterparts.

While organic foods aren't perfect, don't despair. There are a few things you can do to avoid the most toxic pesticides without breaking your budget.

— *Eat local.* The first thing I would recommend is to eat locally grown foods purchased at a nearby farmers' market. Since the produce hasn't traveled across the world, it'll be fresher and more nutritious than foods that took weeks to get to the grocery store.

— *Avoid the most pesticide-laden produce.* Buying only organic foods is great, but it can be cost prohibitive. No matter what, be sure to avoid the worst offenders. The Environmental Working Group website (www.ewg.org) annually updates what the group calls the "dirty dozen," the 12 foods that contain the most pesticides. On the 2015 list are strawberries, peaches, nectarines, apples, potatoes, grapes, sweet bell peppers, imported snap peas, celery, spinach, hot peppers, and kale or collard greens.

— *Wash fruits and veggies before eating.* When you do buy conventionally grown foods, don't settle for a quick rinse with water. Create a simple spray in a 3:1 ratio of water to vinegar. Just coat your veggies, then rub and rinse with clean water.[14] You can also buy specialized products, such as Fit Organic Fruit & Vegetable Wash, to remove the impurities from your produce.

Change 3: Avoid Excess Sugar

Sugar is everywhere. It is highly addictive and leads to long-term health problems. Because eating sugar creates cravings for more, kids get hooked on sweet processed foods and refined carbohydrates. What's more, sugary drinks and sweet (or starchy) foods can cause changes in the palate and make children less tolerant of foods with sour or bitter flavors, as well as more prone to dislike vegetables and to perceive fruits as less sweet.

If you're a parent who's been trying to get your child to eat less sugar, you already know how challenging it is. It's there at social gatherings, at school, at the bank. It even comes with kids' meals at restaurants. Adults delight in plying children with sugary treats, and kids love it too. But when sugar is so ubiquitous, it adds up quickly in the diet, so much so that the average American eats about 20 teaspoons of added sugar *each day!*[15]

Where the heck is all this sugar coming from? An obvious source in children's diets is soda and store-bought juices. Letting kids drink soda, juice, flavored water, or vitamin water increases their desire for more sweet drinks. The body is unable to perceive and thus regulate the calories consumed from a sugary beverage, so kids don't compensate for any additional drink calories by eating less food calories, and thus weight gain ensues.[16]

Not all sugars are bad. It naturally occurs in fruits and vegetables in the form of fructose, but when you eat them, you're also getting enzymes, vitamins, minerals, and other healthy stuff. A medium-size apple has 19 grams of sugar, and a banana has 14 to 19 grams, depending on how ripe it is. If kids got their sugar solely from fruits, it wouldn't be that big a deal, but sugar makes its way into even savory products to make them more pleasing to the palate.

Added sugar in the form of evaporated cane juice, high-fructose corn syrup, and beet sugar is ubiquitous in processed foods. It's often hidden in foods that you wouldn't assume would contain it. For example, in jarred spaghetti sauce, sugar is often the second ingredient after tomatoes! Most nonfat and low-fat yogurts marketed to kids are loaded with sugar, an average of four teaspoons per four-ounce serving. Can you imagine putting four teaspoons of sugar into a half-cup of yogurt? I'm not suggesting that you never allow your child to eat sugar, but it's important to limit his overall intake. It will not make him feel deprived. Avoid making sweet desserts, like ice cream, a regular nightly ritual.

At my house, we make our own treats so that we can use the highest-quality ingredients while avoiding artificial additives and unnecessary sugar. Having to make them ourselves limits how often we eat them. When we do have a dessert, it's usually a fruit cobbler, an apple pie, cookies, or muffins. Richer desserts and cakes are savored on rare occasions and birthdays, which makes them truly special treats!

TCM Wisdom for Eating Healthy

Now that you're familiar with the red-, yellow-, and green-light food system, it's time to return to Traditional Chinese Medicine for more guidance on how to support your child with food. In TCM dietetics, it is recommended that children eat at regular intervals. Not going too long or too short between meals is a way to support the Earth Element. The digestive system needs to fill up and then empty before taking in the next meal, so constant snacking is hard on a child's Earth Element.

It's important that children fill up at each meal with green-light foods that nourish their bodies. When a child is eating lots of red- and yellow-light foods, she's constantly hungry, not only because those foods are addicting, but also because they're lacking in important nutrients.

Another important tenet in TCM dietetics is avoiding too many cold and raw foods. To understand why, imagine that there is a "digestive fire" in your body that cooks the food you eat. It dampens the digestive fire to consume too many cold or raw foods, such as iced drinks or veggies or yogurt straight out of the fridge, and this makes it less effective at breaking food down into the nutrients needed to nourish the body. I don't think it's realistic for kids—or anyone, for that matter—to eat all cooked foods, but I do think a healthy mix of cooked, warm foods along with raw foods is a balanced way to eat so as not to dampen the digestive fire.

My top tips for eating healthy according to TCM are:

- Eat at regular intervals and avoid snacking all day.
- Chew food well.
- Be present during mealtime; avoid watching TV or reading a book.
- Moderately cook foods, such as by steaming or sautéing.
- Avoid using too many ingredients in each meal.

In addition to the red-, yellow-, and green-light system, eating for your element is something to consider. It involves taking elemental imbalances into consideration, adding foods that support the Dominant Element, and eating for the season. (The food lists that follow are commonly known in TCM to support each element and are based on *Healing with Whole Foods* by Paul Pitchford.[17])

Most important, pay careful attention to how your child's body reacts to foods because that will let you know if you're on the right nutritional track. Make sure to use your common sense, too. For example, if your child complains of a stomachache after eating certain foods, try an elimination diet with each food in question to see if it's triggering a reaction. In Chapter 6, I'll outline the steps for doing an elimination diet.

When using the Five Elements to heal with foods, you'll choose your foods in the following order:

- Foods for the element that is most out of balance
- Foods for the current season and/or foods for your child's Dominant Element

How you choose the foods to support elemental healing really will depend on your child's situation. You'll want your child to eat supportive foods in Step 1 for several months to promote healing. But you will also have to take into account the season and what's available in your area, so Steps 1 and 2 may be combined as needed to help your child achieve a well-rounded diet.

- *Step 1: Provide foods that support the most out-of-balance element.* From Chapter 3, you may have found an imbalance in one of your child's elements that is contributing to a health problem. Eating certain foods can help bring the element back into balance. For example, if Earth is out of balance, your child should avoid cold, iced, and raw foods. Even in the summer, this would mean skipping iced drinks, frozen foods like Popsicles, or really cold foods like smoothies. Instead, have him eat fruits and vegetables at room temperature, and lightly sauté vegetables or other foods like apples or spinach. In this way, you can prepare foods that his body will more easily assimilate.

- *Step 2: Provide in-season foods that support your child's Dominant Element.* Consider your child's Dominant Element along with what foods are in season. For example, a Fire child generally needs more cooling foods, but as the weather gets colder in the fall, he will need to add more neutral and warming foods to his diet. A Fire child in the fall would be best supported by adding a moderate amount of sour foods into his diet, such as sauerkraut, olives, pickles, leeks, adzuki beans, or green apples.

Wood Element

Foods that *support* the Wood Element include:

- Moderately spicy foods, such as:
  - Chives
  - Watercress
  - Leeks
  - Onions
  - Rosemary
  - Basil
- Bitter foods, such as:
  - Lettuce
  - Asparagus
  - Kale
  - Cabbage
  - Quinoa
  - Amaranth
  - Chamomile tea
- Dark-purple and red fruits and vegetables, such as:
  - Beets
  - Blackberries
  - Blueberries
  - Goji berries
  - Lychees
  - Quince
  - Plums

Foods that *deplete* the Wood Element include:

- Foods high in saturated fats
- Hydrogenated oils
- GMO oils like corn, soy, cottonseed, and canola
- Nuts and seeds (in excess of 2 ounces daily)
- Any processed or refined foods
- Sodas and energy drinks

Wood is associated with the season of *spring*. During spring, these foods are recommended:

- Green foods
- Baby greens (lettuce and field greens)
- Sprouted grains
- Vegetables
- Legumes
- Other complex carbohydrates

Fire Element

For the Fire Element, foods can be particularly healing, and those rich in calcium promote calm, clarity, and better sleep. Fire children should eat foods that promote calcium absorption.

Foods that *support* the Fire Element include:

- Reishi mushrooms
- Mulberries
- Lemons
- Raw or low-temperature-pasteurized cow's milk
- Goat milk
- Ghee
- Foods rich in calcium and magnesium, like:
  - Dark, leafy greens
  - Brown rice
  - Cucumber
  - Apples
  - Cabbage
  - Fresh wheat germ
  - Wild blue-green algae

Foods that *deplete* the Fire Element include:

- Heavy and rich foods
- Meats
- Eggs
- Nuts, seeds, and grains (when overconsumed)

***Summer* is the season of Fire, the hottest season of the year. Fresh foods that have a cooling nature are recommended, such as:**

- Tomatoes
- Apples
- Watermelon
- Grapes
- Cucumber
- Raspberries
- Lemons
- Limes
- Mint
- Chamomile, peppermint, and chrysanthemum teas

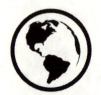

Earth Element

Foods that *support* the Earth Element include:

- Carbohydrate-rich vegetables, such as:
  - Winter squash
  - Pumpkin
  - Carrots
  - Turnips
  - Rutabagas
  - Sweet potatoes
  - Yams
  - Garbanzo beans
  - Black beans

- Vegetables that have a strong taste, such as:
  - Onions
  - Leeks
  - Fennel
  - Garlic
  - Ginger
  - Black pepper
  - Cinnamon
  - Nutmeg

- Small amounts of unrefined sweeteners, such as:
  - » Molasses
  - » Rice syrup
  - » Barley malt
  - » Cherries and dates (to flavor and sweeten foods)

Foods that *deplete* the Earth Element include:

- Too many cold, raw, or iced foods and drinks
- Citrus fruits
- Sprouts
- Raw spinach
- Raw chard
- Tofu
- Sugar
- Dairy products

Late *summer* is the season associated with the Earth Element. During late summer, focus on foods that are gold, orange, or round, especially:

- Carrots
- Turnips
- Yams
- Sweet potatoes
- Squash
- Peas
- Millet

- Corn
- String beans
- Cabbage
- Garbanzo beans
- Apricots
- Cantaloupe

Metal Element

To alleviate the dry skin often associated with the Metal Element, the best foods are carrots, winter squash, pumpkin, broccoli, parsley, kale, turnips, and watercress.

Other foods that support the Metal Element include:

- Sweet rice
- Oats
- Sweet potatoes
- Mustard greens
- Molasses
- Rice syrup
- Poached pears with cinnamon and honey

- Strong, spicy foods like:
  - Chilies
  - Garlic
  - Ginger
  - Horseradish
  - Green onion (the white part)
  - Radishes, including Daikon
  - White peppercorns

Foods that *deplete* the Metal Element include eating too many:

- Meat and dairy products
- Processed foods
- Fried and greasy food
- Raw or iced food
- Citrus juices
- Refined white salt

***Fall* is the season of Metal. Beneficial foods for fall include:**

- Sauerkraut
- Olives
- Pickles
- Leeks
- Green onions
- Adzuki beans
- Sea salt
- Rose hip tea
- Vinegar
- Lemons
- Limes
- Grapefruit
- Green apples

Water Element

Water is the most complex element of the Five-Element system. It has a dual nature of both hot and cold, which coexist in homeostatic balance. When they are out of balance, symptoms may be present with either a cold or hot nature. The foods for this section focus on conditions where cold predominates; thus warming and mildly warm spices are used. When cold wanes and heat predominates, the opposite treatment principle is applied, with recommended foods similar to those that support the Fire Element.

Foods to *support* the Water Element include:

- Walnuts
- Almonds
- Black sesame seeds
- Fenugreek seeds
- Anise seeds
- Cloves
- Black peppercorns
- Dried ginger
- Cinnamon
- Black beans
- Quinoa
- Chicken
- Lamb
- Trout
- Salmon
- Raspberry leaf tea
- Parsley
- Ghee

***Winter* is the season of the Water Element. During winter, your child should eat salty and bitter foods, as well as:**

- Lettuce
- Watercress
- Endive
- Escarole
- Turnips
- Celery
- Alfalfa
- Rye
- Oats
- Quinoa
- Amaranth
- Millet
- Barley
- Miso
- Soy sauce
- Sea salt

Now go to Appendix C and add healing foods to your child's healing program. Write down any foods you'd like to incorporate into her diet to help heal an elemental imbalance, foods you'll incorporate for the current season, and foods to support her Dominant Element.

CHAPTER SIX

Find the Hidden Food Triggers Making Your Child Sick

What if, by simply changing what your child eats, you can get rid of annoying chronic symptoms? It really can be *that* simple. What I've seen time and time again is that after removing an offending ingredient, a child is often symptom-free or dramatically improved! When I'm working with kids who have chronic issues such as environmental allergies, eczema, asthma, hyperactivity, anxiety, stomachaches, or any other digestive symptoms, the first thing I look at is their diet.

Food triggers can cause both chronic and acute symptoms in children, especially the kind of symptoms that aren't solved by pharmaceuticals and don't respond to normal treatments. A food trigger is an allergy, intolerance, or sensitivity to a food that causes an adverse reaction in the body—anything from hives and ana-phylaxis to chronic runny nose, cough, ear infections, stomach-aches, loose stool, nausea, constipation, or diarrhea.

This chapter will explore food triggers, their causes, corre-sponding symptoms, and how to heal their effects. We'll start by exploring the differences among the three types of food triggers, then shift the focus to two: food intolerances and sensitivities.

The Three Types of Food Triggers

Food allergies are immune reactions in which the body produces a blood protein called an IgE antibody in response to certain foods. IgE antibodies attach themselves to a type of white blood cell called a mast cell, which releases prostaglandins and other chemicals that are responsible for things like increased mucus production, nasal congestion, hives, swelling, breathing difficulties, and anaphylaxis. According to the FDA, there are more than 160 foods that cause allergic reactions, but 90 percent of food allergies are due to only eight: milk, eggs, fish, shellfish, tree nuts, peanuts, wheat, and soy.[1] Children with allergies generally need to avoid the offending foods for the rest of their life, although sometimes allergies do lessen with age.

Food intolerances are due to an error in the way the body processes a food, but they are not actual rejections of the food by the immune system. Food intolerance reactions are usually milder than allergies and often involve irritation of the stomach. Common symptoms of food intolerances are gas, bloating, abdominal cramping, nausea, heartburn, headaches, and irritability.

Intolerance to lactose, a milk sugar found in dairy products, is very common. When a person is lactose intolerant, he lacks the enzymes to digest the lactose sugar in dairy products. Because the lactose isn't properly broken down, it causes painful gas, abdominal cramping, and diarrhea. If your child has regular stomachaches, start a food diary or simply pay attention to see if there is a pattern with dairy consumption. Note that sometimes, symptoms of intolerances are unnoticeable when the food is present in small amounts but very uncomfortable once a high enough quantity is eaten.

Food sensitivities aren't as straightforward as food allergies or intolerances. Essentially, a particular food will cause an adverse reaction in the body, but unlike a food allergy, there's no single set of symptoms. Within the holistic medical community, it is believed that food sensitivities are often linked to an immune response associated with IgG antibodies (as opposed to the IgE antibodies of an allergy response). There is still much debate in the Western medical community as to whether this is a reliable test of food sensitivity. However, many doctors and health practitioners find a high correlation between symptoms related to eating foods that produce a higher IgG response and a resolution of those symptoms when the offending foods are eliminated.

While food allergies require an immediate response, intolerances and sensitivities are easy to miss because the adverse reaction is often delayed. When a person has an allergic reaction, it's a very convincing reason to avoid the food. But when the dairy eaten at breakfast is causing a runny nose the next day, it's not immediately apparent that you have a food sensitivity.

Do You Really Need to Investigate Food?

Because they're not easy to identify, food triggers are often dismissed out of hand. We don't usually think of food triggers causing anything but digestive symptoms, but they can also cause behavior and mood issues, sleep problems, congestion, runny nose, and ear infections. Food triggers also lead to inflammation, which makes conditions like asthma and eczema worse.

Resistance to the idea of food triggers is very common, and doctors rarely address food sensitivities as a cause of illness. Parents often don't want to go down the rabbit hole of research because it seems scary and overwhelming to change their children's diets, especially if their pediatricians aren't particularly supportive. But you can also look at it this way: If food is the problem, then it's something that *you* can manage because what you feed your child is under your control. So there's something concrete you can do about your child's symptoms—and that's very good news!

Many parents whom I've worked with have already tried eliminating suspect foods from the diet and found no change. However, it's easy to make mistakes in an elimination diet that can lead to false negative results.

- *Mistake 1: Not being diligent enough about avoiding trigger foods.* If a suspected trigger food is only partially eliminated from a child's diet, then it isn't a true elimination diet. For example, if you are trying to test dairy, an innocent dollop of sour cream on a taco can cause symptoms up to several days after it is eaten.
- *Mistake 2: Not sticking with it long enough.* If a trigger food is completely eliminated, but for too short a time, say for only three or four days, the body won't have a chance to heal so there's little, if any, change in symptoms.
- *Mistake 3: Eliminating only one suspect food.* If a child has multiple food sensitivities such as gluten, dairy, *and* eggs, then removing only one of those foods from the child's diet may not cause significant improvement.

To properly test for a food trigger, you must eliminate *all* suspected food(s) *100 percent* from the diet for at least *two weeks* to give the body a chance to become more balanced.

Causes and Symptoms of Food Intolerances

In addition to foods, you can be intolerant to compounds and chemicals in the food, including:

- Sugars: lactose, sucrose, maltose
- Artificial colors such as tartrazine (FD&C #5) and other azo dyes
- Artificial flavorings
- Preservatives
- Histamines
- Tyramine
- Salicylates
- Benzoates

- BHA and BHT
- Sulfites
- Monosodium glutamate (MSG)

Common responses to these compounds include skin reactions such as hives, diarrhea, constipation, nausea, stomach upset, asthma, chest tightness, facial numbness, tingling in the limbs, hyperactivity, lightheadedness, dizziness, headaches, nasal congestion, swelling, and migraines.[2]

When I first started working with Annie, an Earth child, she got horrible stomach cramps that were so painful they'd wake her up at night. I noticed that if she ate too much cheese or ice cream, she'd get urgent diarrhea or a stomachache, and I suspected she had a dairy intolerance. Her body doesn't have the enzymes to properly break down the lactose sugar in milk, and as the undigested milk sugar travels through her digestive system, her body has an upset reaction. Once we eliminated dairy, her stomach cramps went away, but if she eats dairy again they come right back—strong evidence that dairy is a food trigger for her.

If you suspect a food intolerance, the best strategy is to confirm it with an elimination diet, then completely avoid the offending food or food chemical. Unfortunately, in most cases there is no cure for food intolerances. For intolerances related to an enzyme deficiency, such as lactose intolerance, supplementing with enzymes, like lactase, can be helpful in preventing or lessening symptoms.

Causes and Symptoms of Food Sensitivities

Food sensitivity symptoms vary greatly, develop gradually, and can get worse over time if untreated. Most people have multiple sensitivities to trigger foods that are common parts of the diet. Symptoms are intermittent and vary in intensity, depending on the quantity of the offending food that is eaten. Food sensitivity reactions are slow and can take anywhere from 4 to 72 hours to manifest, which often masks the identity of the offending food.[3]

Two kids may have a sensitivity to the same food yet manifest completely different symptoms. One child eating gluten may get a headache while another might get chronic nasal congestion. Without a single, clear-cut mechanism triggering the adverse reaction, food sensitivity is easy to dismiss as the cause of chronic, low-grade symptoms.

The food trigger of my son Noah, a Metal child, used to cause red, dry, bumpy eczema all over his body. After trying a gluten- and dairy-free diet, his skin actually got much worse. Working with his holistic pediatrician, we did some food-sensitivity testing and learned that eggs were his biggest trigger. Suddenly it all made sense. When I took Noah off gluten and dairy, everything I made was loaded with eggs, so of course his skin worsened. Since Noah was a super-picky eater at the time, it took about four months before he was off eggs completely, but once we managed to eliminate them, his skin improved dramatically.

One theory about the cause of food sensitivities is that there is a failure to activate the gut immune system at birth, which leads to severe imbalances in the Earth and Metal Elements. Anything that interferes with normal, healthy gut flora—such as formula feeding; too-early introduction of solids to an immature gut; or eating too many red-light foods, GMOs, and chemicals—can lead to food sensitivities. Prolonged stress, flu, severe illness, traveler's diarrhea, or digestive trauma such as a surgery, bowel blockage, or even food poisoning can also be causes.

Symptoms of food sensitivity include digestive illness, frequent illness, repeated infections, excess phlegm production, cough, sore throat, throat clearing, sticky and red or swollen eyes, depression, anxiety, mood disorders, hyperactivity, lack of focus, migraines, headaches, dizziness, sleeping problems, hives, eczema, dry or itchy skin, shortness of breath, and chest tightness. Children with food sensitivities often have dark circles under their eyes and a tired look despite getting plenty of sleep. In babies, food sensitivities may present as colic, stomachaches, and failure to thrive. Food sensitivities are often associated with ADHD, autism, learning problems, and behavioral problems, but the symptoms improve when trigger foods are eliminated from the diet. If your child is under- or overweight, food sensitivities should also be investigated.

Food Triggers and the Five Elements

From a TCM perspective, food sensitivities are due to an imbalance in the Earth Element. That's why, in children, we always want to nurture and support the Earth Element; it's vital to a child's overall health. Depending on the element affected, food sensitivities will create differing but specific symptoms. If a child has food sensitivities, there is always an imbalance in the Earth Element, but that doesn't mean he'll always have obvious digestive problems.

- If the Wood Element is affected, symptoms such as headaches, migraines, dizziness, lightheadedness, blurry vision, hyperactivity, and irritability are likely.
- If the Fire Element is affected, then the child may have symptoms such as hives, flushing of the face, mood disorders, anxiety, sleeping problems, hyperactivity, or impulsivity.
- If just the Earth Element is affected, a child will have digestive problems such as constipation, diarrhea, loose stool, nausea, vomiting, gas, bloating, and fatigue.
- If the Metal Element is affected, he'll have dry skin, eczema, runny nose, cough, congestion, frequent illness, asthma, or allergies.
- If the Water Element is affected, a child will feel "out of it" and have symptoms of depression, low energy, lack of focus, low appetite, stiff or achy joints, and dark circles under the eyes.

How to Treat Food Sensitivities

Food sensitivities can be treated if an elimination diet is followed and the gut is allowed to repair itself. It can take anywhere from 3 to 12 months, depending on the severity of the condition and how much the gut was impacted. During the healing period, it is necessary to continue to avoid the trigger foods completely. If the child has a tiny bit, it won't set her back too much, but if she is still eating a trigger food several times a week, it's going to interfere with gut function.

Healthy gut flora need to be restored during this healing period. Daily probiotics will help repopulate the gut with beneficial bacteria and strengthen the ecological barrier of the intestines. This process takes six to eight weeks, depending on the state of one's gut permeability and gut flora. You can support this process further by adding in lacto-fermented foods and beverages. Have your child consume homemade broths and gelatin to heal and seal the gut. Most important, eliminate red-light foods, reduce yellow-light foods, and increase green-light foods.

Below, I outline four steps you can take to diagnose food triggers, but there's no single correct way to go about it. It depends on how bad the symptoms are, how picky your child is, what other testing has already been done, and your own observations about your child's reactions to certain foods. Start with either Step 1 or 2—you may already suspect a food and want to jump in with an elimination diet, or you may want to contact your doctor for tests. With my son Noah, we started with an elimination diet, but because he got worse on the elimination diet, we opted for testing as our second step. Do what makes sense for your child's situation; however, if she is having a severe reaction to food, contact your doctor for allergy testing.

If you need guidance, reach out to a pediatric acupuncturist or other health practitioner who can guide you on the best course of action for your child. To find one in your area, please visit www .kidsloveacupuncture.com/directory.

Step 1: Elimination Diet

— Begin with simple observations. Start a food journal to track your child's diet and reactions. See if you can find a correlation between certain foods and symptoms of ill health.

— For two weeks, remove the foods from your child's diet that you think are the most likely triggers. I typically suggest starting with dairy and gluten unless the parents have observed a pattern of sensitivity reactions that point to other foods. (For instance, if a parent sees that her child gets a rash when he eats eggs, the first thing they need to do is eliminate eggs.)

The six most common trigger foods are gluten, dairy, eggs, nuts, soy, and corn. If you can eliminate all six, that will give you the best results, but if that proves too difficult, start with just gluten and dairy. If symptoms don't alleviate, then eliminate two other foods and so on until you test all of them.

During this period, try to eliminate common food chemicals that many kids are intolerant to, such as artificial colors and flavors, preservatives, and additives. (For a full list, see Appendix E.)

Know that after eliminating an offending food, there's typically a healing crisis where the child feels worse for two to five days. Then they feel significantly better by day six or seven, so you use the second week to calm the body's reaction further.

— After the two-week (or three-week) elimination period, reintroduce foods one at a time, every two to three days. (This interval allows for you to note both immediate and delayed symptoms of a food trigger.) If your child has a clear reaction to an item, immediately stop giving her the food, then pause a few days before introducing another new food. Remember, adverse reactions can be anything from fatigue, irritability, and sleep problems to runny nose, congestion, throat clearing, headaches, stomachaches, hyperactivity, impulsivity, and nausea.

— If you find your child has a food trigger, remove the offending items from your child's diet completely for 3 to 12 months. (See Step 3 for more details.) Don't be tempted to continually test the trigger food to see if there's still a reaction; every time you do this, you're actually impeding your child's healing.

I understand that when a food trigger doesn't cause an anaphylactic reaction, it's harder for some people to accept that it exists. You may get flak from people who don't understand what you're doing or why it's important. With my own kids, I found it easier to just say they had food allergies rather than explain intolerances and sensitivities; family, teachers, and other caregivers then took it more seriously. Over time, you'll find suitable replacements for food triggers that your child will enjoy. It will become part of your lifestyle, and you will learn to work around those trigger foods.

An elimination diet is helpful, but there may be challenges if your child has multiple sensitivities, your family eats out a lot, or your child is extremely picky. If you're eliminating foods containing gluten, dairy, and corn and those are the majority of the foods your child eats, it can be very difficult to even get your child to eat during the testing period. So if you're struggling to remove trigger foods from your child's diet, it may be best to opt for testing.

Step 2: Testing

There are several ways to test for a food sensitivity: IgG food antibody tests; the ALCAT test, which checks for white blood cell response to foods; or a skin patch test to check for non-IgE delayed food reactions.

IgG food sensitivity testing can be prescribed by an acupuncturist or holistic practitioner. If these tests show that your child has food sensitivities, proceed to Step 3, and be sure to eliminate the offending foods from the diet. However, if you start with testing as your first step, you can also confirm the results with an elimination diet before moving on to Step 3, so you and your child can see the benefits for yourself.

If testing shows your child has multiple or numerous food sensitivities, it may be unrealistic to avoid them all. Instead use an elimination diet to determine which food triggers cause the most severe reactions, and then limit and rotate the lesser trigger foods.

If the results of the IgG and ALCAT tests are negative but you still suspect food is triggering your child's symptoms, you can try a skin patch test. While the skin patch test is done by an allergist, not all allergists offer it, so be clear what you want when making an appointment. The skin patch test checks for non-IgE-mediated delayed food reactions. For this test, the foods your child eats on a regular basis are pureed and placed in contact with the skin for 24 hours to see if a reaction is triggered. This test has been helpful for determining delayed-response food triggers in several of my patients.

When Joey came to me, he'd been having chronic diarrhea, slow weight gain, and painful diaper rash for four months. After extensive medical testing, including an endoscopy and colonoscopy, doctors were no closer to figuring out what was causing Joey's diarrhea. We tried an elimination diet and found lactose and sugars to be his triggers. Removing these foods improved, but didn't eliminate, Joey's diarrhea. A skin patch test showed that he was having delayed reactions to blueberries and avocados—two foods that he ate frequently! Once those foods were eliminated, his stools returned to normal and he began gaining weight again.

Unfortunately, none of these tests are a guaranteed way to figure out your child's food triggers. Testing is not infallible, and there can be false negatives. The most reliable indicator of a food trigger is *the body's reaction to the food,* so it's important to always do your own qualitative investigation and track your child's symptoms to see if you can connect them to a food he is eating.

Step 3: Heal the Gut and Balance the Earth Element

Now that you know your child's food triggers, you'll want to remove them from the diet completely for a minimum of three months. With some foods, like gluten and dairy, it can take 9 to

12 months for the gut to completely heal. You must also heal the Earth Element. The Earth Element is responsible for proper digestion of food, and when out of balance it can cause food sensitivities. Here are the steps to take:

- Supplement with probiotics. (For more information, visit www.robinraygreen.com/probiotics.)
- Add more cultured foods to the diet.
- Avoid using medications unless medically necessary.
- Avoid artificial colors and flavors, preservatives, and other food additives.
- Avoid fast food and junk food (red-light foods).
- Eat organic whenever possible.

Step 4: Food Challenge

Once you've eliminated the trigger foods for several months, it's time to do a food challenge. You'll reintroduce triggers and check for adverse reactions to see if the foods will continue to cause problems.

Now, this doesn't mean you should revert to your child's previous diet and hope for the best. Instead, just as with the elimination diet, reintroduce foods one at a time every two or three days unless you witness a reaction. If the child has a clear reaction to a food, then you want to give it a few more days before you challenge him with any other foods.

If any of the foods are still a problem after the food challenge, continue to exclude them from the diet for a few more months before attempting another food challenge. If you find your child doesn't react to the foods, that's great news! You can let your child eat the food in small amounts, but be sure to rotate foods and not allow former triggers to become mainstays in the diet. For instance, Noah can now eat gluten and dairy without getting eczema. However, we still choose to keep them mostly out of his diet. We typically eat gluten and dairy only on special occasions or when we're eating out.

What If You Don't Find a Trigger?

If you strictly followed all four steps above and saw no changes, it could be that food is not a trigger. Your child's gut might have a severe imbalance that needs deeper healing, especially if he has a chronic condition or digestive problems. You may need guidance from an acupuncturist or holistic doctor. Also consider the GAPS Introduction Diet outlined in Dr. Natasha Campbell-McBride's book *Gut and Psychology Syndrome.* The GAPS Introduction diet is helpful in cases where deeper gut healing is needed. And check out the Recommended Resources for other books, websites, and acupuncturist recommendations.

If you find that your child does have a food trigger, be sure and address it in your healing plan in Appendix C.

CHAPTER SEVEN

Balance the Five Elements with Massage and Acupressure

This chapter is intended to guide parents who wish to aid their child's healing and alleviate elemental imbalance with hands-on intervention. You will learn how acupressure and a special type of Chinese pediatric massage called *tuina* (pronounced "twee-nah") can be used to promote elemental balance and treat your child's symptoms.

Tuina and acupressure are safe and effective and can be used in conjunction with Western medical treatments. While acupressure is fairly well known, tuina massage is largely unknown in the West, and it is my sincere hope to change that!

The Basics of Tuina Massage

Tuina has been around for over 3,000 years. It is appropriate for both children and adults, and I have used it on my own children and almost every child I treat in my practice. Tuina feels wonderful, and most kids enjoy it. Sometimes it tickles a little, so kids may laugh while you're doing it. In fact, a few kids in my practice refer to it as the "tickle massage"; by the end of their sessions, even the parents are giggling—a child's laughter is so contagious! Laughter in itself is very healing and has a positive effect on everyone.

Just as a baby's and toddler's nervous system and circulatory system are not fully mature, neither is their meridian system. Special techniques, such as tuina, were developed to tap into a child's immature meridian system in a gentle and restorative way. This is why tuina massage is most effective for children under the age of 5, although it can be used in children through age 12. In general, I recommend acupressure for children over 6.

If you are performing tuina on a baby, you may need a partner to hold or distract him during the massage. You can also gently massage your baby while he sleeps. Hand and finger massage are easiest to do on napping infants.

Tuina is a way to connect with your child's body, mind, and spirit. In TCM, it is believed that your loving and healing intentions are transferred energetically to your child. This energy transfer strengthens your bond and promotes deep connection. I've seen some pretty miraculous healing from parents who lovingly and regularly perform tuina massage. In fact, I have hundreds of testimonials from parents who were able to treat their child's cough, asthma, conjunctivitis, sleeping problems, and more with these simple massage techniques.

Word of Caution

Do not perform tuina massage or acupressure over cuts, abrasions, open wounds, severe eczema, cysts, or tumors. Please be cautious if you child is taking heavy medications. If your child has a spinal cord injury and cannot give you feedback, use only the lightest, gentlest touch.

This type of massage is safe, effective, and totally natural. It can be used in conjunction with medications and medical procedures. However, as powerful as this massage is, it cannot replace medications, such as fast-acting asthma inhalers, for acute symptoms.

Massage Setup and Techniques

Don't let tuina's simplicity fool you. These are powerful techniques, but there are a few pointers you'll need to get right in order for it to be effective. Before you begin, remember to:

1. Trim your fingernails and file the edges smooth so you don't accidentally scratch your child.

2. Find the right massage medium to put on your hands and the child's skin such as cornstarch-based baby powders, massage oil, or lotion. Make sure whatever you use is free of chemicals and fragrances. I suggest olive oil, apricot kernel oil, jojoba oil, or coconut oil. Consider patch testing, if you've never used the product before. (Apply a small amount on the inside of the elbow, and check for reactions 24 hours later.)

3. Make sure the room where you'll be working is warm so your child doesn't get cold during the massage.

There are special techniques that differentiate tuina massage from a Swedish-type massage, in which muscles are mostly kneaded. With tuina massage, you'll be stroking, pushing, pulling, and pressing various points on the body. These movements should be gentle yet firm, even and rhythmic.

Most tuina massage techniques will be performed from 50 to 300 times in very rapid succession. It's such a fast movement that I have found it easier to time the massage on certain points rather than to count how many strokes I've used. For example, if I massage the pointer finger, I know 20 seconds is about 100 strokes.

Use firm pressure, but also be loving and gentle. Always check in with your child's comfort and stay in tune with her body language. If she fusses or cries out, reduce the pressure being used, change the spot you're working on, or position her differently to make her more comfortable. Talk soothingly to her and tell her how great she's doing; never get mad or punish her during massage. Encourage an older child to speak up; ask her how she likes the pressure and make sure she is comfortable with giving feedback.

Chinese Wellness Massage: The Basic Protocol

This wellness massage incorporates tuina techniques and can be used on all kids up to the age of 12. It is the basic protocol you'll use as a starting point for balancing your child's element. It is based on Fan Ya-Li's book *Chinese Pediatric Massage Therapy*, but I've adapted it here with my own descriptions and photos. (For a free massage companion kit and to watch a video of how to do these techniques, please visit www .robinraygreen.com/healyourchild.)

The wellness massage consists of five massage techniques that are performed successively. You can do the techniques in any order. However, when all five are done together they have a cumulative effect that strengthens the effectiveness of the overall massage. For elemental balancing and support, perform the entire massage once a day. After the massage, you may want to add a couple of acupressure points specific to your child's elemental imbalance or health problem.

1. Spinal Roll Back Massage

This massages the muscles next to the spine along the entire back and has specific therapeutic effects depending on which part of the spine it is focused on. When focused on the back from the base of the shoulder blade to the base of the neck, it will help stimulate all the acupuncture points associated with the lungs and chest. If you're unable to perform the full wellness massage, do just the Spinal Roll; it is one of the quickest and most powerful ways to massage the acupressure points for all elements.

To perform this massage, focus on the muscle tissue on both sides of the spine. Gently but firmly "pinch" the muscle tissue between your thumb and forefinger. As you push your thumbs forward up the spine, continue to pull down and pinch the muscle tissue. This should produce a pleasant feeling of pressure as you roll up the back to the top of the shoulders. (See Figures 7.1 and 7.2.)

Do this massage for 10 to 60 seconds, or until the skin turns pink.

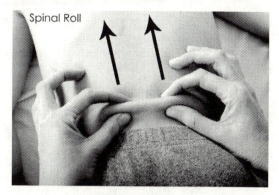

Figure 7.1

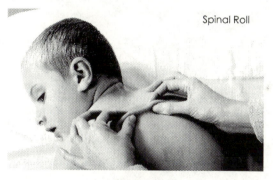

Figure 7.2

2. Circle Rubbing on the Palm

This is a general technique for harmonizing and balancing all the elements. It can be used for almost every condition your child may have, because it helps to restore balance and strengthen the body overall. You only need to perform this massage on one hand. Oil is very helpful here for preventing chafing, especially if your or your child's hands are moist.

Look at the palm of your child's hand and see how the inner portion forms a depression. Using your thumb, rub in circles along the outer border of this depression. If rubbing the left palm, use a clockwise motion; if rubbing the right palm, use a counterclockwise motion. (See Figure 7.3.)

- For up to 2 years: Rub 100 times (20 sec)
- For 2–5 years: Rub 200 times (40 sec)
- For 6–12 years: Rub 300 times (60 sec)

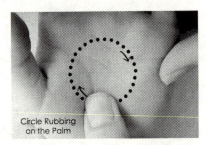

Circle Rubbing
on the Palm

Figure 7.3

3. Line Pressing on the Thumb

This technique helps balance your child's Earth Element, supports the entire digestive system, and promotes overall wellness. Even if you don't have an Earth child, massaging this point is beneficial because a healthy Earth Element is key to robust health and a strong immune system.

Start at the lateral or outer part of the thumb next to the tip of the fingernail, and rub downward toward the base of the thumb pad where it meets the wrist. (See Figure 7.4.) When you get to the wrist, lift and repeat. (See Figure 7.5.)

- For up to 2 years: Rub 100–200 times (20–40 sec)
- For 2–5 years: Rub 200–300 times (40–60 sec)
- For 6–12 years: Rub 500 times (90 sec)

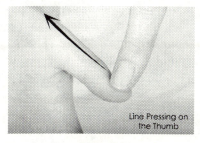

Figure 7.4

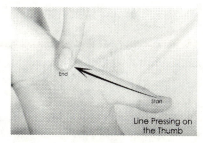

Figure 7.5

4. Circle Rubbing on the Abdomen—Clockwise

This massage supports overall digestive function and elimination and balances the Earth Element, the foundation of a healthy immune system. It helps ensure that qi is flowing evenly throughout the abdomen and intestines.

Rub the abdomen around the belly button in a clockwise direction with your four fingers or the palm of your hand. (See Figure 7.6.)

- For up to 2 years: Rub 100 times (20 sec)
- For 2–5 years: Rub 200 times (40 sec)
- For 6–12 years: Rub 300 times (60 sec)

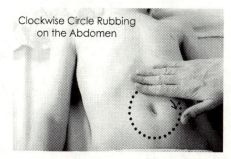

Figure 7.6

5. Kneading Stomach 36 Acupressure Point

This acupressure point is essential in any wellness massage. It helps boost energy, assists digestive function, and supports healthy immune function. It is also traditionally used to treat nausea and stomachaches.

Starting at the outside of the leg just above the ankle, run your finger up the leg until it falls into a dip in the muscle tissue located about three finger-widths (your child's fingers) below the bottom of the kneecap. (See Figure 7.7.) This is Stomach 36 (ST-36). If you need help finding this point, you can also watch the Chinese Wellness Massage Video at www.robinraygreen.com.

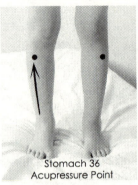

Stomach 36
Acupressure Point

Figure 7.7

- For up to 2 years: Rub 100 times (20 sec)
- For 2–5 years: Rub 300 times (60 sec)
- For 6–12 years: Rub 500 times (90 sec)

Elemental Balancing with Finger Tuina

To balance your child's element, a simple tuina finger massage can be done anytime and anyplace. Finger tuina can be used to balance the Dominant or Influential Element. It can also be used to treat any one of the Five Elements that is out of balance and triggering symptoms. If you're not sure which elements need balancing or support, be sure to take the Five-Element Diagnostic Test in Appendix B.

With your child's hand palm up, simply press in a line along the finger corresponding to the element you want to balance:

- The thumb corresponds to Earth.
- The pointer finger corresponds to Wood.
- The middle finger corresponds to Fire.
- The ring finger corresponds to Metal.
- The pinkie finger corresponds to Water.

If you need to support and strengthen a *deficient* element, start from the tip of the finger and press toward the base, then rapidly lift and repeat.

If you need to calm an *excessive* element, start from the base of the finger and press toward the tip, then rapidly lift and repeat.

For example, if you have an Earth child who has frequent colds and a chronic runny nose, that means the Metal Element is deficient. To balance Metal, rapidly massage the ring finger by pressing in a line from the tip of the finger to the base.

- For up to 2 years: Rub 100–200 times (20–40 sec)
- For 2–5 years: Rub 200–300 times (40–60 sec)
- For 6–12 years: Rub 500 times (90 sec)

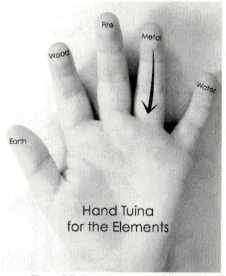

Figure 7.8: Supporting a Deficient Water Element with Finger Tuina

Acupressure for Elemental Imbalances

Acupressure has an even longer history than pediatric tuina; it has been around for over 5,000 years.[1] While tuina uses methods unique to children's growing bodies, acupressure points can be used for any age and are located on the same meridians used to perform acupuncture. The main difference, of course, is that pressure rather than needles is applied to the point.

Acupressure is safe and effective, and you can do it anywhere because no special tools are required. I encourage parents to use acupressure not only to balance the elements but also to treat specific symptoms. According to acupressure expert Michael Reed Gach, "Acupressure can be effective in helping relieve headaches, eyestrain, sinus problems, neck pain, backaches, arthritis, muscle aches, and tension due to stress."

Because acupressure points use the TCM meridian system, you may find that you need to treat a specific ailment at a site that is distant from the problem. This is because the most powerful points on the meridian are often located below the elbows and knees; working on them will affect the meridian related to the problem.

Acupressure can be safely used to augment any Western medical treatments your child is currently undergoing. However, acupressure cannot replace proper medical care. If your child suffers from a serious physical, mental, or emotional condition, be sure to seek medical care from a qualified doctor or health practitioner.

Guidelines for Acupressure

Each acupressure point is found by looking and feeling for anatomical "landmarks." As you search for the point with your fingers, often you'll sense a change in the way the muscle tissue feels. You may detect a knot or tightness or a dip in the muscle tissue that creates a bit of a hollow. The pictures in this chapter will help guide you to the point, and then your fingers will help you find the location more specifically on your child's body.

Many parents I've worked with are concerned that they're doing it wrong, but you don't have to be! Acupressure is fairly forgiving, so even if you're not exactly on a point, you'll probably get close enough to the meridian for the pressure to still be effective. The sizes of the points vary—some are about the size of a quarter, while others are around the size of a dime.

While there are several acupressure techniques, I find that firm pressure, or firm pressure with kneading, is the easiest way to stimulate the acupressure points on children. The amount of pressure is not related to how effective the session will be; while the pressure should be firm, it should *not* cause any pain. The optimal level of pressure will be different for each child, and each area of the body will have a different sensitivity and require a different amount of pressure.

When you first touch an acupressure point, start with light pressure, then gradually increase it. You'll then hold the point with firm pressure for 10 to 60 seconds, depending on the child's age:

- For up to 12 months: 10 seconds
- For 1–2 years: 20 seconds
- For 2–4 years: 30 seconds
- For 5–6 years: 40 seconds
- For 6 years and up: 50 seconds or more

What follows is a description of how to balance each element and treat the specific health conditions that show up when that element is out of balance. You can use the described acupressure points in combination with the wellness massage or on their own to treat specific health problems.

Wood

The pointer finger represents the Wood Element. Balance the Wood Element with finger tuina, pressing in a line from the base of the pointer finger to the tip. Because the Wood Element is rarely in a deficient state, you will not massage Wood from tip to base, which is the direction you would massage to strengthen a deficient element. Instead, if you do find your child's Wood Element deficient, you need to nourish Water, which in turn nourishes Wood. To nourish Wood, massage the pinkie finger from tip to base.

When the Wood Element is out of balance, a child may have symptoms such as anger, irritability, headaches, migraines, muscle spasms, irritated eyes, or eyestrain. To treat these symptoms and concurrently balance the Wood Element, apply acupressure first to point Liver 3 (LV-3) and then Large Intestine 4 (LI-4).

LV-3 is located on the top of the foot between the first and second toes, level with the end of the first metatarsal, or big toe bone. (See Figure 7.9.)

LI-4 is located on the web of the hand between the thumb and pointer finger in the middle of the pointer finger metacarpal bone. (See Figure 7.10.)

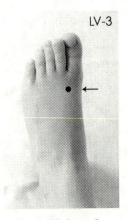

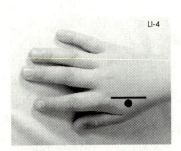

Figure 7.9: Liver 3   *Figure 7.10:* Large Intestine 4

Fire

The middle finger represents the Fire Element. When the Fire Element is deficient, there will often be symptoms such as light sleep, anxiety, insomnia, hypoglycemia, or mild moodiness. Strengthen Fire by pressing in a line from the tip of the middle finger to the base. If the Fire Element is excessive and your child is experiencing extreme mood swings, volatile temper, red cheeks, impulsivity, and hyperactivity, then balance the excess Fire Element by pressing in a line from base to tip.

Heart 7 (HT-7) is a powerful acupressure point for supporting Fire and calming the mind from worries, anxiety, stress, distract-edness, fears, restlessness, or moodiness. In addition, HT-7 can help treat insomnia and poor sleep when due to a Fire imbalance.

HT-7 is located on the wrist crease, in line with the pinkie. (See Figure 7.11.)

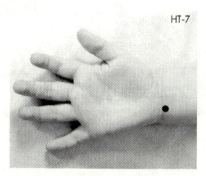

Figure 7.11: Heart 7

Earth

In finger tuina, the thumb and thumb pad correspond to Earth. Whether the Earth Element is deficient or balanced, you can strengthen it by pressing in a line from the tip of the thumb to the base of the thumb pad. When Earth is deficient, your child will have symptoms of low appetite, loose stools or diarrhea, weak muscles, bloating, or low energy. If Earth is excessive and the child has symptoms of overeating, bloating, or indigestion, you can balance Earth by massaging from the base of the thumb pad to the tip of the thumb.

Acupressure at Spleen 6 (SP-6) has a balancing effect for symptoms of Earth imbalances listed above. In addition, SP-6 has a calming effect on the mind, so it is good for children with anxiety that affects their stomach. To strengthen the effects of SP-6, especially for stomachaches with poor digestion, add the Conception Vessel 12 point (CV-12), which is often used in combination for these symptoms.

SP-6 is located on the inside of the lower leg, about three finger-widths from the midpoint of the malleolus, or ankle bone, in line with and just below the edge of the tibia, or leg bone. (See Figure 7.12.)

CV-12 is located on the abdomen, midway between the belly button and where the ribs meet at the sternum. (See Figure 7.13.)

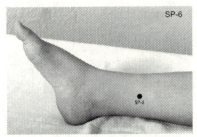

Figure 7.12: Spleen 6

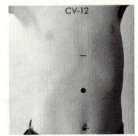

Figure 7.13: Conception Vessel 12

Metal

The ring finger represents Metal. When Metal is in a deficient state with symptoms such as frequent illness, chronic runny nose, dry skin, or year-round allergies—or even if this element is balanced—strengthen it by pressing in a line from the tip of the ring finger to the base. When Metal is excessive and there are symptoms of strong and loud cough, seasonal allergies with itchy red eyes and nasal congestion, asthma, or eczema, balance Metal by pressing from the base to the tip of the ring finger.

Acupressure at Lung 7 (LU-7) is great for cough, asthma, and lung problems such as bronchitis. When combined with Large Intestine 20 (LI-20), it can be used to treat runny nose, nasal congestion, sinus infections, and frequent colds.

You can find LU-7 by following the thumb up the wrist just past the bony prominence of the radial bone. (See Figure 7.14.)

LI-20 is on the face next to the nose at the level of the nostril. (See Figure 7.15.)

LU-7

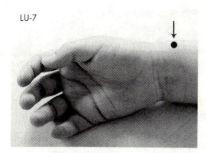

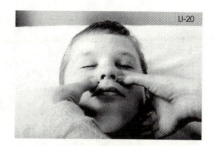

Figure 7.14: Lung 7

Figure 7.15: Large Intestine 20

Water

The pinkie finger represents Water. When the Water Element is balanced, you can further strengthen it by line pressing from the tip of the pinkie to the base. If your child's Water Element is deficient, you can use the same technique for symptoms such as low motivation, low energy, backaches, poor teeth or bone development, tendency toward ear infections, dark circles under the eyes, delays in meeting developmental milestones, slow growth, or bedwetting. If Water is excessive, the child will have symptoms like ADHD with predominant inattention, trouble focusing, difficulty completing tasks, kidney stones, or repeated urinary tract infections. For an excess Water Element, press in a line from the base of the pinkie to the tip.

While acupressure at Kidney 3 (KI-3) can be used to correct any type of Water imbalance, it is particularly helpful for deficient Water issues. KI-3 is located on the inside of the ankle, midway between the ankle bone and the Achilles tendon. (See Figure 7.16.)

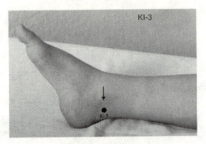

Figure 7.16: Kidney 3

Auriculotherapy and Ear Seeds to Balance the Elements and Treat Symptoms

Auriculotherapy is another way to support healing, address symptoms, and restore balance to the elements. You can think of it as reflexology for the ear. The ear represents a map, or microsystem, of the entire body. Certain spots on the ear correspond to areas of the body, symptoms, and the organ networks corresponding to the Five Elements. For at-home auriculotherapy, you apply pressure to corresponding points with a special ear probe, a toothpick, or ear seeds.

Ear seeds are tiny vaccaria seeds that have been placed on a piece of self-adhesive tape. When applied to special points on the ear, they provide gentle and continuous pressure that stimulates healing. Simply apply the ear seed to the area you want to treat and leave it for 24 to 48 hours. You need to apply pressure to only one ear at a time, so you can alternate which ear you do with fresh seeds. (**Caution:** Do not apply ear seeds on babies or children younger than age three. Do not leave ear seeds on your child's ear or body for longer than 48 hours.)

Auriculotherapy has been used for thousands of years around the world for conditions such as sleep problems, cough, asthma, rhinitis, earache, stomachache, constipation, and hyperactivity. What I love about auriculotherapy is that if you use ear seeds to do it, they work in the background as your child goes about her normal routine. Most kids think they're fun.

To find the appropriate auriculotherapy points, look at Chart 7.1 and find the spots related to the elements that need balancing. You can use a probe or a toothpick to check for tenderness, markings, or discoloration in the parts of the ear that correspond to the element you want to treat. For example, a child with a Wood imbalance may have a vein or light spot around one of the ear's inner furrows. (You can also apply ear seeds to any of the acupressure points previously discussed.)

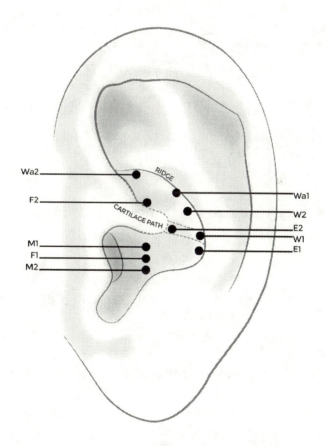

Associated Element and TCM Organ Network	Location of Auriculotherapy Point
Wood (W1): Liver	Under the ridge at the highest point
Wood (W2): Gallbladder	Under the ridge on the back wall
Fire (F1): Heart	Center and deepest point
Fire (F2): Small Intestine	Above cartilage path in curve
Earth (E1): Spleen/Pancreas	Under the ridge, just under the end of the cartilage path
Earth (E2): Stomach	Right past the tip of the cartilage
Metal (M1): Lungs	Right above the center and deepest point
Metal (M2): Lungs	Right below the center and deepest point
Water (Wa1): Kidney	Under the ridge at the highest point
Water (Wa2): Bladder	Under the ridge near the front of the ear

Chart 7.1: Auriculotherapy Points

You can purchase a special ear seed kit for kids with further information about particular auriculotherapy points at www .robinraygreen.com/earseeds. For a variety of kits and options, visit www.earseeds.com.

Now it is time to go into your healing plan in Appendix C and do the following:

- Write down the finger tuina massage and the direction you'll need to press to balance the necessary elements. Remember: If balanced or deficient, strengthen by pressing from the tip of the finger to the base. If excessive, press from the base to the tip of the finger.
- Write down the acupressure points you can use to treat the element that is out of balance or the symptoms your child is experiencing.
- Write down the auriculotherapy points you can apply pressure or ear seeds to.

For more information and videos on tuina massage and acupressure, visit www.robinraygreen.com.

AFTERWORD

The Five-Element approach to healing has been around for thousands of years, and it works because it goes beyond the linear model of addressing illness. It's a complete holistic approach that helps you understand who your child is and then discover the imbalances that are creating issues. Then you can create a healing program that includes natural remedies, dietary changes, lifestyle changes, and massage to support your unique child.

Along the journey, you'll need to trust the process—healing from the inside out requires work! Change isn't always easy, but it's totally worth it when you see your child grow stronger and more resilient. I invite you to trust that even simple remedies can be powerful! The most important thing you can do when trying a remedy or making a change is to be consistent and allow time for healing to occur. Trust that your child's body can heal itself. Most importantly, trust your own instincts about what your child needs when it comes to his health care.

The healing program you create is not set in stone; rather, it's a starting point for working toward resolving your child's challenges and focusing on bringing out the best in your child. You are beginning a dynamic process that will change as you make your way through the steps. Take small, but consistent steps toward adjusting your family's diet and lifestyle and before you know it you'll look back and be amazed at how far you've come.

If you need more support, ideas, and resources for implementing your child's healing program, please join me and the 5-Element Way community at www.robinraygreen.com as well as Facebook.com/AuthorRobinRayGreen.

APPENDIX A

Five-Element Questionnaire

How to Take the Questionnaire

This questionnaire is designed to help you identify your child's Dominant and Influential Elements according to the Five-Element system in Traditional Chinese Medicine. To determine your child's Dominant Element, check the questions that apply to your child on a regular basis. Think about how your child acts across multiple settings such as school, social gatherings, sporting events, and home as you check off the characteristics that resonate with your child's way of being in the world.

Because your child comprises all five elements, it's normal to check off characteristics under all five. But you'll find the majority of your child's characteristics will fall under one or two of the elements. After completing the questionnaire, read through Chapter 2, paying particular attention to the elements for which your child has the highest scores, to glean more insight into your child's Dominant Element.

Wood Element

❑ Energetic, always on the go since a very early age
❑ Curious about how things work
❑ Likes adventure and exploration
❑ Seeks movement and stimulation
❑ Has an intense, driven personality
❑ Wants to figure out how to do it herself
❑ Pushes rules and boundaries and tests limits
❑ Enjoys overcoming obstacles and challenges
❑ Goal oriented, goes all out to win and dislikes losing
❑ Enjoys being the leader in a group
❑ Shows great determination and perseverance
❑ Argumentative and tenacious when she thinks she's right
❑ Athletic, with high physical endurance/stamina
❑ Tends to get angry or frustrated easily
❑ May resist authority figures, like teachers, parents, etc.
❑ May not filter thoughts; communication may be blunt or hurtful to others
❑ Can forget polite manners (saying please/thank you)
❑ Competitive, often attracted to team sports
❑ May have loud and frequent outbursts of anger or strong emotion
❑ Gets bored easily
❑ Has trouble sitting still or staying in seat during class
❑ Figures out things through logic
❑ Energy level is super active compared with that of other kids; has a ton of energy
❑ Motivated to compete and win
❑ Emotional response to stress is anger, frustration, or quick temper

Total Number Checked ＿＿＿＿＿＿

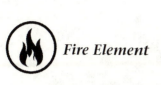 *Fire Element*

- ❏ Loves being the center of attention
- ❏ Enjoys entertaining others—singing, dancing, acting, telling jokes
- ❏ Charismatic, charming, friendly, and enthusiastic
- ❏ Easily makes friends
- ❏ Comfortable in a variety of social settings
- ❏ Recharges by being around and talking to others
- ❏ Very sensory aware—enjoys touching different textures, playing with colors
- ❏ Intuitive learner, or learns best through music, games, and play
- ❏ Masters tasks quickly and is ready to move on to the next thing
- ❏ Sensitive to others' emotions, thoughts, feelings
- ❏ Can be moody and dramatic
- ❏ Can be impulsive, or impulsively touches, pulls, or picks at things
- ❏ Can have a hard time finishing projects if bored or if a skill is mastered
- ❏ Seeks attention, acknowledgement, and approval from parents and others
- ❏ Lives in the moment and doesn't always consider consequences (as appropriate for age)
- ❏ When upset, tends toward dramatic outbursts of emotion
- ❏ Can have trouble falling or staying asleep
- ❏ Is easily overstimulated by television and video games; has a hard time winding down afterward
- ❏ Gets flushed face or blushes easily
- ❏ Does things fast—thinking, talking, moving, eating
- ❏ Easily gets hot or sweats

- ❏ Restless, has a hard time relaxing
- ❏ Is very active; has lots of energy compared with other kids
- ❏ Motivated by being the star, being adored, having fun, and experiencing new things
- ❏ Emotional response to stress is anxiety or overexcitement

Total Number Checked _____

🌍 *Earth Element*

- ❏ Loves being in a group setting
- ❏ Enjoys talking to people and making friends
- ❏ Is a natural caregiver or little mother/father
- ❏ Gets upset or worried if others are upset or arguing
- ❏ Outgoing, but doesn't want to be the center of attention
- ❏ Enjoys helping out
- ❏ Enjoys singing and humming
- ❏ Cares deeply about family, friends, caregivers, and pets
- ❏ Very affectionate—loves to hug, kiss, or be physically close to parents, especially mother
- ❏ Attached to parents, teachers, and caregivers; can have separation anxiety
- ❏ Can get distracted in class due to chatting with or helping others
- ❏ Is easygoing and goes with the flow
- ❏ Sensitive to others' emotions and feelings
- ❏ Gets overwhelmed by details
- ❏ Craves sweets and white foods like bread, crackers, and potato chips

- ❏ May soothe emotions through eating, or eats when bored
- ❏ Enjoys eating, cooking, or exploring new foods
- ❏ Worries can lead to nausea or stomachaches
- ❏ Can struggle with obesity or being overweight
- ❏ May have difficulty voicing her needs
- ❏ Learns through context, connections, and relationships
- ❏ Tends to mull things over for a while before making a decision
- ❏ Motivated by pleasing others
- ❏ Energy level can range from very active to active, but needs quiet time
- ❏ Emotional response to stress is overthinking, worrying, or having obsessive thoughts

Total Number Checked _____

Metal Element

- ❏ Sweet, gentle, and easygoing, but also has stubborn side
- ❏ Can see the big picture, but also all the details
- ❏ Slow to warm up in social settings, but then friendly
- ❏ Prefers routines and rhythms in daily life
- ❏ Enjoys completing tasks and checking things off a list
- ❏ Likes to keep belongings and toys fairly organized (for his age)
- ❏ Love for logic, patterns, and puzzles
- ❏ Will follow the rules; you don't have to tell him twice
- ❏ Doesn't like to get in trouble
- ❏ Sensitive to the environment and others' emotions
- ❏ Feels things deeply; can be easily embarrassed

❏ Gets upset when routines are disturbed, or doesn't like change

❏ Will try really hard and wants to "do it right"

❏ May have perfectionist tendencies

❏ Can be stubborn and unbending when his mind is set on something

❏ Gets upset when others break the rules or don't follow along

❏ Can get hyperfocused on a task and gets behind on schoolwork

❏ Is sensitive to tastes, smells, and textures—may be a picky eater

❏ Tends to cry or become upset if corrected or punished

❏ Is sensitive to the clothing on his body if it doesn't feel right, such as being bothered by a shirt tag

❏ Tends toward colds, coughs, or dry or rough skin, especially in the fall

❏ Tends to have a softer voice than other children

❏ Active, but enjoys quiet time

❏ Motivated by pleasing authority figures

❏ Emotional response to stress is tears, negative thoughts, or fixation on mistakes

Total Number Checked _____

Water Element

❏ Mellow, mild-mannered, goes with the flow

❏ Easygoing, less demanding

❏ Quiet, prefers to be in the background of activity

❏ Attracted to deep thoughts and philosophy, even at a young age

❏ Has a deep inner strength or wisdom beyond her years

❏ Can be reasoned with, since she craves wisdom/knowledge

❏ Enjoys magic, mythology, and mystical ideas, books, and games

❏ Innovative; thinks outside the box

❏ Very imaginative—can have a very rich inner world

❏ Learns well using imagination—making up stories, creativity, inner exploration

❏ Can become withdrawn and depressed

❏ Can be stubborn at times

❏ Often does not have an appropriate sense of time and dislikes being rushed

❏ Can harbor deep fears

❏ Takes a while to warm up to people outside of family and close friends

❏ Often quiet and contemplative, sometimes withdrawn

❏ Prefers to stay at home and needs alone time after school or social activities

❏ Easily overwhelmed by lots of noise and other environmental stimuli

❏ Advanced emotional intelligence; feels deeply

❏ Excels in a flexible environment with less structure

❏ Quiet in class, may go unnoticed by teacher

❏ Tends to have a rounder body shape

❏ Energy level is somewhat active, but needs alone time

❏ Motivated by a deeper understanding of why or how she benefits

❏ Emotional response to stress is to withdraw, run away, hide, or create imagined stories about the stressor

Total Number Checked _____

List the Elements with Highest Scores:

1.

2.

3.

Which one do you think is your child's Dominant Element? Which one do you think is your child's Influential Element? Go back to Chapter 2 and read through the element descriptions.

APPENDIX B

Five-Element Diagnostic Test

The Five-Element Diagnostic Test is designed to help you identify any elemental imbalances your child may have that are contributing to her health challenges. Some symptoms may show up in multiple categories as they may be related to imbalances in more than one Element. After finishing the diagnostic test, you should be able to see which elements overall are out of balance.

For this test, you'll rate symptoms on a scale of 0 to 3. By applying a rating of severity, you'll get a more accurate score that reflects the health of each element. Apply your rating to symptoms that your child currently has, or those she's had in the past that tend to recur. Don't rate symptoms that have appeared in the past, but haven't occurred since. You'll be able to best help your child if you focus on her current symptoms and patterns.

Rating Scale

0 = Never
1 = Mild
2 = Occasional or Moderate
3 = Frequent or Severe

WOOD

Excess:

_____ Headaches, especially at the temples
or top of head

_____ Migraines

_____ Muscle spasms

_____ Red, irritated eyes

_____ Restlessness, difficulty sitting still

_____ Heartburn, ulcers

_____ Uncomfortable or foul-smelling gas

_____ Oily, acne-prone skin

_____ Irritability, frustration

_____ Quick temper and/or angry outbursts

_____ Defiance

_____ Hyperactivity

_____ Impulsive behavior

_____ Irritable bowel syndrome

Score _____

Deficiency:

_____ Fatigue

_____ Eyestrain

_____ Blurry vision

_____ Insomnia, difficulty falling asleep, or light sleeping

_____ Environmental or food allergies

_____ Food intolerances

_____ Difficulty digesting gluten/dairy

_____ Nausea or vomiting, especially when upset

_____ Painful gas

_____ Depression with anger and frustrated feelings

_____ Tendency to bruise

Score _____

FIRE

Excess:

_____	Overexcitement
_____	Anxiety or panic
_____	Dread or fear
_____	Tendency to blush, flushing
_____	Sweating
_____	Sores on mouth, lips, or tongue
_____	Rashes, hives
_____	Speech problems such as stuttering or difficulty with articulation
_____	Insomnia, excessive dreaming, nightmares, restless sleep
_____	Mood swings, quick temper
_____	Inability to think straight, feelings of being overwhelmed, difficulty making decisions
_____	Hyperactivity
_____	Impulsivity

Score _____

Deficiency:

_____	Tiredness, lack of stamina
_____	Lack of focus, distractibility
_____	Feelings of being scattered or overwhelmed
_____	Mental and emotional disorders
_____	Forgetfulness, confusion
_____	Light sleep that's easily disturbed by ambient sounds
_____	Sweating, spontaneous sweating
_____	Fears of rejection and other phobias
_____	Need for adoration and friendship
_____	Poor circulation
_____	Anemia

Score _____

EARTH

Excess:

_____ Digestive problems, especially gas, bloating, constipation

_____ Recurrent abdominal pain or stomach upset, ulcers

_____ Low or high blood sugar

_____ Overweight, obesity

_____ Emotional eating, overeating

_____ Nausea or vomiting

_____ Thick mucus in sinuses

_____ Headache with heavy feeling, related to worry or conflict

_____ Heaviness in the head or limbs

_____ Weak joints

_____ Tiredness, difficulty getting started

Score _____

Deficiency:

_____ Constant hunger, overeating

_____ Craving for sweets after meals

_____ Low appetite

_____ Belching

_____ Hiccups

_____ Tooth decay

_____ Soft muscles or poor muscle tone

_____ Sugar cravings

_____ Easily tires, lack of endurance

_____ Loose stools or diarrhea

_____ Nervous stomach leading to urgent bowel movements

_____ Overthinking, racing thoughts

_____ Worry

_____ Self-esteem issues

Score _____

METAL

Excess:

_____ Stiff muscles, lack of flexibility

_____ Hypersensitivity to taste, touch, smells, and sounds

_____ Easily triggered gag reflex

_____ Dry skin, hair, nails

_____ Acute eczema, rashes, or hives

_____ Chronic stuffy nose

_____ Shortness of breath, wheezing

_____ Cough, croup, stridor

_____ Asthma

_____ Allergies

_____ Sinus problems

_____ Ear infections

_____ Enlarged tonsils

_____ Constipation with dry stools

Score _____

Deficiency:

_____ Chronic food and environmental allergies

_____ Colds that rapidly go to chest

_____ Frequent illness or upper respiratory tract infections

_____ Chronic runny nose

_____ Chronic eczema and/or psoriasis

_____ Irritable bowel syndrome

_____ Tendency to get infections—sinus, skin, nose, chest

_____ Sensory processing disorders

_____ Dry nose or mouth

_____ Throat clearing

_____ Weak or soft voice

Score _____

WATER

Excess:

———— Difficulty falling asleep

———— Fears, especially fear of the dark

———— Bladder infections

———— Kidney stones

———— Hypersensitivity to light and loud sounds

———— Coarse or brittle hair

———— Tendency to be frightened, excessive fears or phobias

———— Lack of appropriate fear

———— Sweating and feeling hot at night

———— Dry nose or throat

Score ————————

Deficiency:

———— Lack of focus, poor memory and retention

———— Disconnection, inattention

———— Cold hands and feet

———— Tendency to tire out, low stamina

———— Need for more sleep than average

———— Bedwetting

———— Delayed milestones

———— Cavities, poor bone or tooth development

———— Backache or knee pain

———— Delayed closure of the fontanelle

———— Hearing problems

———— Genetic conditions (all)

———— Cognitive impairment

———— Dark circles under the eyes

Score ————————

List the two elements that had the highest scores. These are the elements you want to focus on rebalancing first.

1.

2.

APPENDIX C

Healing Program Template

You can come to this Appendix at any point as you read through the book. I've created this template to help you collect and organize the important information that pertains to your child's healing program.

First, you'll write down the things you already know from your child's current and past medical history and issues you'd like to address. Then you'll add your child's Dominant and Influential Elements, along with any elemental imbalances that need to be addressed. Finally, you'll write down the changes you plan to make to your child's diet, lifestyle, routines, schedule, and so on. At the end, list your top three priorities and work on implementing those first.

You do not have to fill out the entire healing program. Write only in the areas where changes need to be made.

Child's Name:_____

Age:_____

Medical Investigations	
Health, Emotional, Behavioral, or Social Challenges	
Medical Diagnosis (if any)	
Past Medical Treatments: What worked? What didn't work?	
Current Medical Treatments	
Possible Future Medical Treatments	
Elemental Patterns	
Dominant Element	
Season of Dominant Element	
Any Symptoms Related to the Dominant Element?	
Influential Element	
Season of Influential Element	
Any Symptoms Related to the Influential Element?	
Elemental Imbalances:	1. 2. 3.

Supporting Your Child's Element and Correcting Imbalances List the things you can do to support your child's Dominant and Influential Elements or rebalance the elements. Write down the easiest and most impactful things you can implement.	
Massage	When will you add massage into your child's routine? Finger Tuina: List which fingers and the direction you'll press (base to tip or tip to base) 1. 2. 3.
Acupressure	Which acupressure points will you massage daily? 1. 2. 3. 4.
Gut Flora	Will you add a daily probiotic to your child's routine? Which one and how will you administer it? (More info at: www.robinraygreen.com/probiotics.)

Food Triggers	Do you need to investigate food triggers? What steps will you take? 1. 2. 3. 4. 5. 6.
Acupuncture/Herbs	Will you seek the care of a pediatric acupuncturist or herbalist? Do you have an herbal remedy reference? What herbs or natural remedies will you try?
Environment	Are there any changes you'll make to your child's living environment? Cleaners Personal care items Food and drink containers Mattress Other items you're bringing into your home

Movement/Activities	Does your child need more or less activity? What will you change in this area?
Screen Time	Is screen time a concern? Do you need to cut back or make changes? How will you reinforce and/or explain these changes?
Sleep	Does your child need a bedtime routine? Sleep support? Nightly massage?
Seasonal Support	In which season(s) do you feel your child needs the most support? How can you support your child during this season? Changes to routine? Diet? After-school activities? Natural remedies?
Stress Management	What practices can you add to your child's routine to help with stress management?
Mindfulness Meditation	How can you teach these practices and incorporate them into your (and your child's) daily or weekly routine? Can you add them to something you're already doing?

Gratitude	How can you incorporate a gratitude practice that feels easy and natural? A blessing before meals? Sharing gratitude at dinner or before bed?
Parenting Changes	Is there anything you need to change in the way you're parenting your child? What changes do you need/want to make in your own diet or lifestyle that will help your child?
Behaviors to Model	Are there certain behaviors you need to model for your child (e.g., flexibility, stress management, gratitude, anger management)?
School	Are there any changes in your child's classroom or school environment that will offer better support?
After-School and Social Activities	Does your child's afternoon schedule support his element? Is there too much or too little activity?

Dietary Changes	
Pantry & Fridge Check	Review the items in your pantry and refrigerator, read the labels, and see whether they fall in the red-, yellow-, or green-light category.
	Which top 10 items will you replace with healthier alternatives:
	1.
	2.
	3.
	4.
	5.
	6.
	7.
	8.
	9.
	10.
	Are there any items you want to throw out today?
	What are the worst red-light foods your child is eating? Can you find a healthier alternative? Will they just be special-occasion foods?
	Are there foods or beverages with artificial colors, flavors, additives, or preservatives that you'll need to replace?

Breakfast	What does your child usually eat for breakfast? What improvements can you make to your child's breakfast to boost nutrition?
Lunch	What does your child usually eat for lunch? What improvements can you make to your child's lunch to boost nutrition?
Dinner	What does your child usually eat for dinner? What improvements can you make to your child's dinner to boost nutrition?
Organics	Which items will you begin to buy organic?
Meal Planning	On which day of the week will you plan meals? Will you use a meal planning service?

Looking at the list above, what are the top three priorities for your child's health?

1.
2.
3.

What can you commit to doing or changing over the next 30 days to help address those top three priorities you have for your child? List the steps here and then write them on your calendar:

Week 1

1.
2.
3.

Week 2

1.
2.
3.

Week 3

1.
2.
3.

Week 4

1.
2.
3.

APPENDIX D

Noah's Sample Healing Program

Name: Noah
Age: 18 months

Medical Investigations	
Health, Emotional, Behavioral, or Social Challenges	*Symptoms:* Redness and areas of eczema can change rapidly. Looks great in the morning and then gets really red by the afternoon and evening. The eczema gets worse if he's teething or is sick.
Medical Diagnosis (if any)	Eczema with red, dry, bumpy patches of skin on all limbs, chest, and face. Has gradually gotten worse since starting at 3 months old.
Past Medical Treatments: What worked? What didn't work?	Hydrocortisone cream, Elidel cream, baths with chlorine bleach — After 6 months of trying various creams, there haven't been any significant changes with these treatments, and his eczema has continued to worsen.
Current Medical Treatments	IgE food and environmental allergy blood test, skin prick test for allergies — All negative for environmental and food allergies
Possible Future Medical Treatments	Find holistic or integrative pediatrician

Elemental Patterns	
Dominant Element	Metal
Season of Dominant Element	Fall

Any Symptoms Related to the Dominant Element?	Skin and immune system are related to the Metal Element. Skin also gets worse when he gets sick.
Influential Element	Wood
Season of Influential Element	Spring
Any Symptoms Related to the Influential Element?	No (A few years later, Noah would develop allergies in the spring)
Elemental Imbalances:	1. Metal 2. Earth

Supporting Your Child's Element and Correcting Imbalances

List the things you can do to support your child's Dominant and Influential Elements or rebalance the elements. Write down the easiest and most impactful things you can implement.

Massage	*When will you add massage into your child's routine?* After bath, before bed: Spinal Roll Finger Tuina: 1. Ring finger—tip to base (Metal) 2. Thumb—tip to base (Earth)
Acupressure	*Which acupressure points will you massage daily?* 1. LI-11 2. LU-7 3. ST-36 4. SP-6
Gut Flora	*Will you add a daily probiotic to your child's routine? Which one and how will you administer it?* Klaire Lab's Therbiotic Complete Powder—⅛ tsp twice daily by putting on the inside of his cheek. (Remember to visit www.robin raygreen.com/probiotics for more info on this step.)

Food Triggers	*Do you need to investigate food triggers? What steps will you take?*
	1. *Gluten and Dairy Elimination Trial:* Results: skin got worse
	2. *IgE Blood Test:* Results: negative for any IgE reactions
	3. *Skin Prick Test:* Results: negative, no reactions
	4. *IgG Food Sensitivity Test:* Results: Positive for eggs, gluten, and dairy. Eggs were the strongest trigger of all foods tested.
	5. Eliminate eggs, gluten, and dairy
Acupuncture/Herbs	*Will you seek the care of a pediatric acupuncturist or herbalist? What herbs or natural remedies will you try?*
	Homeopathics:
	Boiron: Sulphur 30X homeopathic remedy 3 pellets 3x/day
	Pekana: Itires 1 drop gradually up to 10 drops/day in water
	Pekana: Renelix 1 drop gradually up to 10 drops/day in water
	Pekana: Apo-Hepat 1 drop gradually up to 10 drops/day in water
	Herbs:
	Chinese Modular Solutions: Harmonize Metal & Wood—for skin and immune system balancing
	Gentle Warriors: Fire Fighter—for skin
	Gentle Warriors: Windbreaker—for respiratory illnesses
	Supplements:
	Fish Oil: Nordic Naturals DHA Jr. 1 tsp/day
	Nordic Naturals GLA oil: ½ tsp/day
	Glutamine: 1000 mg/day
	Quercetin: 450 mg/day

Environment	*Are there any changes you'll make to your child's living environment?*
	Added air filter in whole house
	Added whole house water filter to remove chlorine
	Added reverse osmosis water filter at sink + manually added minerals back into water with Energetix: Spectra-Min
	Cleaners: Switch to DIY vinegar and essential oil cleaners, start using Fragrance Free Detergent by 7th Generation.
	Personal care items: Get rid of all harsh detergents and chemical ingredients. Switch to California Baby brand and ACURE brand
	Food and drink containers: Get rid of all plastic and switch to stainless steel and glass containers and water bottles
	Mattress: Wrap Noah's mattress with wool blanket
	Toys: Get rid of plastic toys, make sure paint on trains is safe
Seasonal Support	*In which season(s) do you feel your child needs the most support? How can you support him during this season?*
	Fall: skin seems to get drier and redder in the fall. Make sure he's getting oils daily.
Mindfulness Meditation	*How can you teach these practices and incorporate them into your (and your child's) daily or weekly routine?*
	Bring back my daily meditation even if it's only for 5 minutes! Stop worrying so much!!!
Gratitude	*How can you incorporate a gratitude practice that feels easy and natural?*
	Focus on gratitude for Noah's overall good health and sweet and happy temperament.

Parenting Changes	*Is there anything you need to change in the way you're parenting your child?*
	Stop focusing on Noah's eczema and start focusing on him as the whole and beautiful child he is. Trust that he will heal and that we'll figure it all out.
	What changes do you need/want to make in your own diet or lifestyle that will help your child?
	I need to stop eating gluten and dairy, too! I know for sure I have trouble digesting dairy. I'm pretty sure gluten is a trigger for me, too.
Dietary Changes	
Pantry & Fridge Check	Start by getting rid of all items with gluten, dairy, and eggs, which includes bread, crackers, yogurt, cottage cheese, bottled salad dressings, and eggs.
	Start reading the labels of EVERYTHING before I buy it!
Organics	*Which items will you begin to buy organic?*
	Anything that Noah will eat!
Meal Planning	*What day of the week will you plan meals?*
	Plan meals on Saturday, batch cook on Sunday.

Looking at this list above, what are the top three priorities for your child's health?

- Getting rid of gluten, dairy, and eggs
- Adding in herbs and supplements
- Doing daily massage and acupressure, twice-weekly acupuncture

What can you commit to doing or changing over the next 30 days to help address those top three priorities you have for your child? List the steps here and then write them in your calendar:

Week 1

- Start trying gluten-free alternatives
- Start trying dairy-free alternatives
- Remove as many foods that contain eggs as is feasible, while still allowing Noah to get enough calories

Week 2

- Try the Sulphur homeopathic remedy for 2 weeks
- Continue finding gluten-, dairy-, and egg-free alternatives
- Daily probiotics and herbs
- Try giving Noah a smoothie with greens in it daily

Week 3

- Purchase gluten- and dairy-free cookbooks
- Search for gluten-, dairy-, and egg-free breakfasts (Hardest meal of the day)
- Try making homemade broth and finger jello from Great Lakes gelatin

Week 4

- Go off of dairy (Noah likes coconut milk! Yay!)
- Continue searching for gluten- and egg-free alternatives to Noah's chicken nuggets
- Start Pekana remedies, since Sulphur homeopathic didn't seem to make any difference

Remember that this is simply one example of one child's healing program. Your child will have his or her own unique journey. Certain categories will be of more or less interest to you based on your child's needs. For instance, there are certain categories that I did not fill out because Noah was a toddler and they didn't apply to him.

APPENDIX E

Common Food Chemicals to Avoid

Here are some commonly found examples of deceptive labeling:

— *All Natural:* Basically anything could have the label "natural" even if there's nothing we could consider natural in it. Here's what the FDA had say about it: "From a food science perspective, it is difficult to define a food product that is 'natural' because the food has probably been processed and is no longer the product of the earth. That said, FDA has not developed a definition for use of the term natural or its derivatives."

— *Natural Flavorings:* The bottom line is there's nothing natural about "natural flavorings." "Natural flavorings" are usually essential oil extracts synthetically made in a lab. While listed as a single ingredient on a label, the term may comprise anywhere from 50 to 100 ingredients, including petroleum-based chemicals and preservatives.

— *Baked with Whole Wheat:* Check the label, because whole wheat may be low on the ingredients list. And if it's not labeled "100% whole wheat," enriched flour is probably the first ingredient.

— *Fresh Baked:* You'll often find this term on breads, rolls, and other baked goods that are treated with dough conditioners. Preservatives are often added to these foods as well to make them look fresh baked while providing longer shelf life.

— *Lean:* This is often used on turkey products like hot dogs, ground turkey, and turkey meatballs. It implies that it's low in fat and healthier for you. Food companies can use this on any seafood or game meat that contains less than 10g total fat, 4.5g or less saturated fat, and less than 95mg cholesterol. "Lean" is not necessarily healthier for you if the animals or fish are farm raised, fed antibiotics, and subjected to inhumane conditions.

— *Sugar Free:* The product may not have sugar, but it probably has artificial sweeteners. My husband once brought home a bottle of barbecue sauce that said "Sugar Free," but it contained aspartame. It's worth reading labels so you don't have to make a trip back to the store!

— *No Added MSG:* MSG stands for monosodium glutamate, and labeling for this chemical has been tricky for years. As consumers began to demand products without MSG, rather than actually remove it from their products, some food companies got around putting it on the label by listing it as a "spice." Some were even so bold as to put "No Added MSG" on the label, even though they knew that MSG was in the ingredients. The FDA finally ruled that companies can't make misleading claims by hiding MSG in the spices or other ingredients. However, the FDA doesn't have the manpower to test all foods to make sure they don't contain MSG. If your child is sensitive to MSG, avoid foods with added "spices," and look on the ingredients list for "free glutamic acid," which is another form of MSG. For a full list of ingredients that contain MSG, visit www.truthinlabeling.org/hiddensources.html.

— *0 g Trans Fats:* Even foods labeled as having no trans fats can actually contain trans fats from hydrogenated oils. According to the FDA, "If a serving contains less than 0.5 gram, the content, when declared, must be expressed as '0 g.'" Just to clarify, that's not the amount in the whole package, but the amount in one serving. So even if you see "0 g Trans Fats" on a label, look at the ingredients list and check to make sure there aren't any hydrogenated oils.

Preservatives and Additives to Look For and Avoid:

Full Name	Abbreviation	What It Does	Found In
tertiary butylhydroquinone	TBHQ	Prevents oils from going rancid, extends shelf life of food	Fast foods, convenience foods
butylated hydroxytoluene, butylated hydroxyanisole	BHT, BHA	Prevents oils from going rancid, extends shelf life of food	Cereals, instant mashed potatoes, chewing gum, dry dessert mixes
Ethylenediamine-tetraacetic acid	EDTA, calcium disodium EDTA, disodium EDTA	Preserves food; promotes color, texture, and flavor	Cereals, cereal bars, snack bars, mayonnaise, canned foods, frozen potatoes
Sulfates, Sulfites		Preserves food, enhances flavor	Dried fruits, prepared fruit and vegetable products
Nitrates, Nitrites		Preserves food, enhances flavor	Cured meats such as hot dogs, lunch meats, pepperoni, salami, bacon
Dimethylpolysiloxane		Added to oils to prevent spattering; added to dry ingredients to prevent clumping	Fast-food oil for french fries, dry gelatin dessert mixes, salt
Propyl gallate		Prevents oils from going rancid	Meat products, microwaveable popcorn, soup mixes, chewing gum, mayonnaise, frozen meals
Perfluorooctanoic acid	PFOA	Surfactant, makes surfaces non-stick	Teflon pans, microwave popcorn bag linings (not listed in ingredients)
Monosodium glutamate and glutamate derivatives	MSG	Enhances flavor, has an addicting quality	Soups, fast foods, processed foods

Full Name	Abbreviation	What It Does	Found In
Carageenan		Thickens, stabilizes, and emulsifies food	Toothpaste, nondairy milks, yogurt, desserts, deli meats
L-cysteine		Conditions dough, increases shelf life and enhances texture of breads, reduces production time	Breads, buns, baked goods, especially at fast-food restaurants
Natural and artificial flavorings		Enhances flavor. Natural flavorings are not "natural" at all, and one may contain 50–100 ingredients, including preservatives.	Fruit juices, prepackaged foods, cereals, sodas, and many other premade foods
Artificial colors (food dyes)		Makes food look more appealing	Crackers, cakes, yogurts, many other products
Bisphenol A	BPA	Hardens plastic	The linings of cans, plastic food containers, other hard plastics

APPENDIX F

Easy Switches to Green-Light Foods

Red- or Yellow-Light Foods	Green-Light Foods
White or wheat bread	Sprouted whole-wheat bread
White pasta	Whole grain and sprouted grain whole wheat pasta, quinoa, and brown rice pasta
Cereal	Whole organic oats or other grains, soaked overnight
Breakfast and cereal bars	Homemade granola bars or trail mix, warm and well-cooked grain cereals and porridge (soaked overnight)
Processed peanut butter sweetned with sugar or high-fructose corn syrup	Freshly crushed peanut butter, sunflower seed butter, or almond butter
Vegetable oils—canola, corn, sunflower, soy	Coconut, avocado, or olive oil
Margarine or substitute butter	Organic butter
Low-fat or nonfat nonorganic milk	Raw or low-temp-pasteurized whole organic milk
Low-fat or nonfat nonorganic yogurt	Whole organic yogurt and sour cream
Nonorganic lunch meats	Organic lunch meats, cooked chicken and meats
Grocery store eggs	Local eggs from pastured chickens
Canned beans	Organic dried beans, soaked then slow cooked
Soy milk, soy protein powder, and most other soy products	Fermented soy such as miso or tempeh
Sucralose (Splenda), aspartame (NutraSweet and Equal), saccharin (Sweet 'N Low), and other artificial sugars	Sucanat, turbinado sugar, raw honey, maple syrup, blackstrap molasses

RECOMMENDED
RESOURCES

Health Resources

Find a Pediatric Acupuncturist

www.kidsloveacupuncture.com/directory

Holistic Health Guides

The Holistic Baby Guide: Alternative Care for Common Health Problems, by Randall Neustaedter

Homeopathic Medicine for Children and Infants, by Dana Ullman

Naturally Healthy Babies and Children: A Commonsense Guide to Herbal Remedies, Nutrition, and Health, by Aviva Jill Romm and William Sears

Smart Medicine for a Healthier Child, by Janet Zand, Robert Rountree, and Rachel Walton

Chinese Medicine and Alternative Health

Between Heaven and Earth: A Guide to Chinese Medicine, by Harriet Beinfield and Efrem Korngold

Fire Child, Water Child: How Understanding the Five Types of ADHD Can Help You Improve Your Child's Self-Esteem and Attention, by Stephen Cowan, M.D.

Healing the New Childhood Epidemics: Autism, ADHD, Asthma, and Allergies: The Groundbreaking Program for the 4-A Disorders, by Kenneth Bock

Healing with Whole Foods, by Paul Pitchford

The Wisdom of Your Child's Face: Discover Your Child's True Nature with Chinese Face Reading, by Jean Haner

Chinese Pediatric Massage and Acupressure

Acupressure's Potent Points: A Guide to Self-Care for Common Ailments, by Michael Reed Gach, Ph.D.

Chinese Pediatric Massage: A Practitioner's Guide, by Kyle Cline, L.M.T.

Chinese Pediatric Massage Therapy: A Parent's and Practitioner's Guide to the Treatment and Prevention of Childhood Disease, by Fan Ya-Li

Resources for Sleep Support

Books and Apps

Meditation Coloring Book: Wonderful Images to Melt Your Worries Away, by Patience Costner

Zentangle. For older kids (ages 10 and up), this is a type of drawing that uses patterns to create art and can be very relaxing and meditative. http://www.zentangle.com

Fragrant Heart. This blog offers free audio meditations and guided relaxations for children. http://www.fragrantheart.com.

Inner Health. This blog offers resources on relaxation and coping skills. The following scripts include guided imagery and can be read to help your child relax. http://www.innerhealthstudio.com/relaxation -scripts-for-children.html

Sleep Meditations for Kids. A smartphone app by Christiane Kerr, produced by Diviniti Publishing Ltd. Helpful for guiding ages 6–12 to relax. Available through iTunes and Google Play.

Online Videos for Relaxation

Guided Meditations for Children - Enchanted Forest, posted on YouTube by Paradise Music. https://youtu.be/b57QvR1Ysyw

Guided Sleep Meditation for Kids and Parents | Relaxation Techniques for Anxiety, posted on YouTube by livewellseries. https://youtu.be/ J6CRlK0zm_Y

Hot Air Balloon Ride: A Guided Meditation for Kids, Children's Visualization for Sleep & Dreaming, posted on YouTube by Sleep Ezy Tonight. https://youtu.be/vlv6Y1tq1sQ

Resources for Healthy Eating and Healthy Guts

Nutrition Guides for Children

Beautiful Babies: Nutrition for Fertility, Pregnancy, Breastfeeding, and Baby's First Foods, by Kristen Michaelis

Super Nutrition for Babies: The Right Way to Feed Your Baby for Optimal Health, by Katherine Erlich, M.D., and Kelly Genzlinger. The authors classify foods according to the four pillars of Weston A. Price and use a similar classification to my red-, yellow-, and green-light foods. However, the four categories they use for food are *Crap, Okay, Pure,* and *Power.*

Guides to Food Allergies and Sensitivities

Dealing with Food Allergies: A Practical Guide to Detecting Culprit Foods and Eating a Healthy, Enjoyable Diet, by Janice Vickerstaff Joneja

Food Allergies and Food Intolerance: The Complete Guide to Their Identification and Treatment, by Jonathan Brostoff and Linda Gamlin

Meal Planning

MOMables. This website has tips for making healthy lunches your child will actually eat. Meal-planning as well as meal-delivery services are offered, with gluten-free and dairy-free options. http://www.momables.com

Naturally Savvy Mom. Real-food meal plans and cookbooks. http://www.naturallysavvymom.com

Real Plans. A meal-planning subscription service that caters to those who want to simplify eating real food. They offer paleo, traditional, and vegetarian meal plans. http://www.realplans.com

Stay Basic. This website helps busy parents eliminate gluten and dairy and create healthy meals. They also offer courses and meal-planning services. http://www.staybasic.com

Cookbooks

The Best Homemade Kids' Lunches on the Planet: Make Lunches Your Kids Will Love with More Than 200 Deliciously Nutritious Meal Ideas, by Laura Fuentes

Bone Broth Secret: A Culinary Adventure in Health, Beauty, and Longevity, by Louise Hay and Heather Dane

Deceptively Delicious: Simple Secrets to Get Your Kids Eating Good Food, by Jessica Seinfeld

Great Food Fast, by Bob Warden

Not Your Mother's Slow Cooker Cookbook, by Beth Hensperger

Nourishing Traditions: The Cookbook That Challenges Politically Correct Nutrition and the Diet Dictocrats, by Sally Fallon and Mary Enig

Slow Cooker: The Best Cookbook Ever, by Diane Phillips

The Sneaky Chef: Simple Strategies for Hiding Healthy Foods in Kids' Favorite Meals, by Missy Chase Lapine

The Vegan Slow Cooker: Simply Set It and Go with 150 Recipes for Intensely Flavorful, Fuss-Free Fare Everyone (Vegan or Not!) Will Devour, by Kathy Hester

Recommended Probiotic Brands

Probiotic brands I recommend can be found online at stores such as http://www.vitacost.com and include:

- Orthomolecular
- Jarrow
- Garden of Life
- Flora

Klaire Labs is another great brand, but you may need to purchase it from a licensed practitioner. For the most up-to-date information on probiotics and recommended brands, visit www.robinraygreen.com/probiotics.

Books on Gut Health and Probiotics

Baby Poop: What Your Pediatrician May Not Tell You, by Linda F. Palmer, D.C.

Cultured Food for Life: How to Make and Serve Delicious Probiotic Foods for Better Health and Wellness, by Donna Schwenk

A Definitive Guide to Gut Bacteria and Probiotics, by Rick Gold

Digestive Wellness: Strengthen the Immune System and Prevent Disease through Healthy Digestion, by Elizabeth Lipski

Gut and Psychology Syndrome: Natural Treatment for Autism, Dyspraxia, A.D.D., Dyslexia, A.D.H.D., Depression, Schizophrenia, by Natasha Campbell-McBride

Resources for Creating a Healthy Home Environment

Environmental Working Group. The group's website lists common chemicals to avoid in food, toys, and personal care products. http://www.ewg.org

Home in Harmony: Designing an Inspired Life, by Christa O'Leary

The Naturally Clean Home: 150 Super-Easy Herbal Formulas for Green Cleaning, by Karyn Seigel-Maier

Resources for Mindfulness and Gratitude

Books to Support Mindfulness

A Handful of Quiet: Happiness in Four Pebbles, by Thich Nhat Hanh and Wietske Vriezen. This is a very simple meditation and the first one that I taught my boys.

Planting Seeds with Music and Songs: Practicing Mindfulness with Children, by Thich Nhat Hanh. The enhanced e-book contains recorded audio music and song lyrics from the book.

Apps to Support Mindfulness

Headspace, by Headspace. This app teaches about meditation through animated videos and has a fun tracking system to encourage kids to meditate daily. Recommended for older children. Available through iTunes, Google Play, and http://www.headspace.com.

Mindfulness for Children, by Jannik Holgersen. This app is great for ages 6–12. It gives kids step-by-step guidance on how to meditate and cultivate mindfulness. Available through iTunes, Google Play, and http://mindful-app.com.

Online Videos for Kids to Practice Mindfulness

Meditation for Kids - The Butterfly - Kids' Meditation, posted on YouTube by OMG. I Can Meditate! https://youtu.be/_mX4JBBIcBk

Mindfulness for Children Free Meditation for Kids, by Jannik Holgersen, posted on YouTube by Mindfulness for Children. This is from the creators of the Mindfulness for Children app. https://youtu.be/SEctySiCol0

Books to Foster Gratitude

Making Grateful Kids: The Science of Building Character, by Jeffrey Froh and Giacomo Bono

Raising Happiness: 10 Steps for More Joyful Kids and Happier Parents, by Christine Carter

Online Videos for Kids to Foster Gratitude

Dealing with Entitled Kids, by Christine Carter, Ph.D., posted on YouTube by Greater Good Science Center. https://youtu.be/IzSfdasZgP0

Tips for Raising Happy Kids, by Christine Carter, Ph.D., posted on YouTube by Greater Good Science Center. https://youtu.be/tKyUidrx0c8

Gratitude - An Inspirational and Stunningly Beautiful Original Short Film HD, posted on YouTube by 4thWeb. https://youtu.be/YCNFnuxhtFM

ENDNOTES

Introduction

1. Delaney, Liam and James P. Smith. "Childhood Health: Trends and Consequences over the Life Course." *The Future of Children* 22.1 (2012): 43-63.

2. "Overweight Prevalence among Children and Adolescents 2011-2012." Centers for Disease Control and Prevention, Center for National Health Statistics, 14 Sep 2014. Web. 4 Jan 2015. http://www.cdc.gov/nchs/data/hestat/obesity_child_11_12/obesity_child_11_12.htm.

3. "Trends in Allergic Conditions among Children: United States, 1997–2011." Centers for Disease Control and Prevention. CDC Center for National Health Statistics, 1 May 2013. Web. 4 Jan. 2015. http://www.cdc.gov/nchs/data/databriefs/db121.htm.

4. "Summary Health Statistics for U.S. Children: National Health Interview Survey, 2012." Centers for Disease Control and Prevention. CDC Center for National Health Statistics, 1 December 2013. Web. 4 Jan. 2015. http://www.cdc.gov/nchs/data/series/sr_10/sr10_258.pdf.

5. Gupta, Ruchi S. et al. "The Prevalence, Severity, and Distribution of Childhood Food Allergy in the United States." *Pediatrics* 128.1 (2011).

6. "Prevalence of Autism Spectrum Disorder among Children Aged 8 Years—Autism and Developmental Disabilities Monitoring Network, 11 Sites, United States, 2010." Centers for Disease Control and Prevention. CDC Center for National Health Statistics, 28 Mar 2014. Web. 4 Jan. 2015. http://www.cdc.gov/mmwr/preview/mmwrhtml/ss6302a1.htm?s_cid=ss6302a1_w.

Chapter 1

1. King, Brian. "Habits of Happy People." Embassy Suites, Monterey. 18 Feb. 2015. Lecture.

2. Lehrer, Paul M., Susan Isenberg, and Stuart M. Hochron. "Asthma and Emotion: A Review." *Journal of Asthma* 30.1 (1993): 5-21. Web.

3. Liangas, G. et al. "Laughter-Associated Asthma." *Journal of Asthma* 41.2 (2004): 217–221. Web.

4. Maciocia, Giovanni. "Diagnosis by Observation." *The Foundations of Chinese Medicine: A Comprehensive Text for Acupuncturists and Herbalists*. 2nd ed. Edinburgh: Churchill Livingstone, 1989. 292.

5. Ibid.

6. Williamson, Marianne. "Day 330." *A Year of Miracles: Daily Devotions and Reflections*. EPub ed. New York: Harper Collins, 2013. 336.

7. Haner, Jean. *The Wisdom of Your Child's Face*. Carlsbad, CA: Hay House, 2010.

8. Ibid.

9. Ibid.

10. Ibid.

11. Ibid.

Chapter 2

1. Cowan, S. *Fire Child, Water Child: How Understanding the Five Types of ADHD Can Help You Improve Your Child's Self-Esteem and Attention*. Oakland, CA: New Harbinger Publications, 2012.

2. Ibid.

Chapter 3

1. Maciocia, Giovanni. "The Five Elements." *The Foundations of Chinese Medicine: A Comprehensive Text for Acupuncturists and Herbalists*. 2nd ed. Edinburgh: Churchill Livingstone, 1989. 26.

2. Loo, May. *Pediatric Acupuncture*. Edinburgh: Churchill Livingstone, 2002. 21.

3. Lichtman, J. et al. "Depression and Coronary Heart Disease." *Circulation* 118 (29 Sept. 2008). Web. 25 Jan 2016. http://circ.ahajournals.org/content/118/17/1768.

4. Loo, May. *Pediatric Acupuncture*.

Chapter 4

1. "National Sleep Foundation Recommends New Sleep Times." National Sleep Foundation, press release, 2 Feb. 2015. Web. 31 Jan. 2016. https://sleep foundation.org/media-center/press-release/national-sleep-foundation -recommends-new-sleep-times.

2. Turnbaugh, P.J. and J.I. Gordon. "The Core Gut Microbiome, Energy Balance and Obesity." *Journal of Physiology* 587 (2009): 4153–4158. doi: 10.1113/jphysiol.2009.174136.

3. Wendelsdorf, Katherine. "Gut Microbes and Diet Interact to Affect Obesity." National Institutes of Health. 16 Sept. 2013. Retrieved April 27, 2015. http://www.nih.gov/researchmatters/september2013/09162013obesity.htm.

4. O'Hara, A.M. and F. Shanahan. "The Gut Flora as a Forgotten Organ." *EMBO Reports*, 7.7 (2006), 688–693. doi:10.1038/sj.embor.7400731.

5. Yano, Jessica M. et al. "Indigenous Bacteria from the Gut Microbiota Regulate Host Serotonin Biosynthesis." *Cell* 161.2 (2015), 264-276.Retrieved 29 June 2015. http://authors.library.caltech.edu/56514.

6. Yano, Jessica M. et al. "Indigenous Bacteria from the Gut Microbiota."

7. O'Leary, Christa. *Home in Harmony: Designing an Inspired Life*. Carlsbad, CA: Hay House, 2014.

8. Sudsuang, Ratree, Vilai Chentanez, and Kongdej Veluvan. "Effect of Buddhist Meditation on Serum Cortisol and Total Protein Levels, Blood Pressure, Pulse Rate, Lung Volume and Reaction Time." *Physiology & Behavior* 50.3 (1991): 543-548. Web.

9. Smith, Jonathan C. "Alterations in Brain and Immune Function Produced by Mindfulness Meditation: Three Caveats." *Psychosomatic Medicine* 66.1 (2004): 148–149. Web.

10. Kabat-Zinn, J. et al. "Effectiveness of a Meditation-Based Stress Reduction Program in the Treatment of Anxiety Disorders." *American Journal of Psychiatry* 149.7 (1992): 936–943. Web.

11. "Christine Carter: Gratitude 365." YouTube video. Greater Good Science Center. Web. 01 Feb. 2016. https://youtu.be/tKyUidrx0c8.

Chapter 5

1. Genzlinger, K. and K. Erlich. *Super Nutrition for Babies: The Right Way to Feed Your Baby for Optimal Health*. Beverly, MA: Fair Winds, 2012.

2. "Any Disorder among Children." National Institute of Mental Health. Web. 01 Feb. 2016. http://www.nimh.nih.gov/health/statistics/prevalence/any -disorder-among-children.shtml.

3. "Press Release." Centers for Disease Control and Prevention. Centers for Disease Control and Prevention, 22 Oct. 2010. Web. 01 Feb. 2016. http://www .cdc.gov/media/pressrel/2010/r101022.html.

4. Boyd, Tim. "Principles of Healthy Diets." Weston A. Price website, 01 Jan. 2000. Web. 01 Feb. 2016. http://www.westonaprice.org/health-topics/ abcs-of-nutrition/principles-of-healthy-diets-2.

5. Genzlinger and Erlich. *Super Nutrition for Babies*.

6. Ibid.

7. Ibid.

8. Boyd, Tim. "Principles of Healthy Diets."

9. Genzlinger and Erlich. *Super Nutrition for Babies*.

10. Franklin, Peter S. et al. "Bread." *Encyclopedia.com*. HighBeam Research, Jan 2003. Web. 1 Nov. 2015. http://www.encyclopedia.com/topic/bread.aspx.

11. "Chorleywood: The Bread That Changed Britain." BBC News, 7 June 2011. Web. 1 Nov. 2015. http://www.bbc.com/news/magazine-13670278.

12. "Food Colours and Hyperactivity." Food Standards Agency. Web. 1 Nov. 2015. https://www.food.gov.uk/science/additives/foodcolours.

13. Jerschow, Elina et al. "Dichlorophenol-Containing Pesticides and Allergies: Results from the US National Health and Nutrition Examination Survey 2005–2006." *Annals of Allergy, Asthma, and Immunology* 109.6 (Dec. 2012), 420-425.

14. Aubrey, Allison. "What Does It Take to Clean Fresh Food?" National Public Radio, 20 Sept 2007. Web. 3 Feb. 2016. http://www.npr.org/templates/story/story.php?storyId=14540742.

15. Erven, Bethene and Cynthia Ogden. "Consumption of Added Sugars among U.S. Adults, 2005–2010." *NCHS Data Brief* 122 (2013 May), 1-8. Web. 1 Nov. 2015.

16. Moss, Michael. *Salt, Sugar, Fat: How the Food Giants Hooked Us.* New York: Random House, 2013.

17. Pitchford, P. *Healing with Whole Foods: Asian Traditions and Modern Nutrition.* Berkeley, CA: North Atlantic Books, 2002.

Chapter 6

1. "Food Allergies: What You Need to Know." U.S. Food and Drug Administration. Retrieved May 31, 2015. http://www.fda.gov/food/resourcesforyou/consumers/ucm079311.htm.

2. Joneja, J.M.V. *Dealing with Food Allergies: a Practical Guide to Detecting Culprit Foods and Eating a Healthy, Enjoyable Diet.* Boulder, CO: Bull Publications, 2003.

3. Brostoff, Jonathan, and Linda Gamlin. *Food Allergies and Food Intolerance: The Complete Guide to Their Identification and Treatment.* Rochester, VT: Healing Arts, 2000.

Chapter 7

1. Gach, M.R. Acupressure's Potent Points: A Guide to Self-Care for Common Ailments. New York: Bantam Books, 1990.

ACKNOWLEDGMENTS

I want to thank so many people who helped make this book possible. First and foremost, I must thank my husband, Dwight, for helping create the space for me to write this book on nights and weekends and all the moments in between. Without him and his witty humor and willingness to pick up the slack, this book would not have made it past the Introduction.

I want to thank my boys, Noah and Nate, for their unwavering faith and constant cheering even when I had to head out to write instead of play! You two are truly my inspirations, and I see many beach trips and play days in our future.

I want to thank my mom for always believing in me and giving me the confidence to pursue my dreams. I want to thank my uncle and aunt, Bob and Lyn, for all your support and for so generously allowing me to use your quiet house and making sure I was well tended to as I wrote!

Thank you to my best friend, Kendra, for always believing that I would become an author even when I didn't! Our conversations helped me work through some of the hardest parts of the book. Thank you Sean Guinan for being my sounding board as I worked out my take on the Five Elements—your support was critical for helping it all gel.

I also owe gigantic thanks to my friend and editor, Michelle Frances, for helping me organize the enormous amount of content that's in this book so that it all makes sense and flows. You are the best book doctor a writer could have!

I want to thank all my patients and their parents for allowing me to include your stories in the book. It's inspiring to work with parents who are so dedicated to helping their kids heal naturally and using TCM to bring out the best in them. Your trust and confidence in me are humbling.

I also want thank the assistants who helped keep my office and my online world running smoothly while I wrote the book: Anita

Silva, Rachel van Dusen, Martha Koch, and Candance Holmes. You are the best!

Thank you, Erin Day Cox, and the ladies in the Enlightened Empire Builders Mastermind: Lindsay Pera, Elena Lipson, Natalie Garay, and Dawn Gibson. Before our retreat I was dangerously close to giving up on this book, and that weekend in Tiburon gave me the boost I needed to fearlessly move forward and submit my book proposal to Hay House. Lindsay, I have so much gratitude for your generous support during all the ups and downs and reminding me to create magic by letting go and allowing things to unfold in their natural order. I want to thank Jen Mazer, the Queen of Manifestation, for helping me to start down this road, to dream big, and to manifest a book published by Hay House!

I want to thank Efrem Korngold, Stephen Cowan, Elisa Song, Jake Fratkin, and Randall Neustaedter for your groundbreaking work with kids and blazing the trail for pediatric acupuncture to go mainstream! In addition, I want to thank the entire acupuncture community along with all the pediatric acupuncturists around the world who have trained with me. Your support and belief in me have helped me build a platform from which to reach parents and truly change lives. Together we are making a difference! A huge blanket of gratitude goes out to all the acupuncturists in the PAC on Facebook who helped inspire ideas and resources for the book.

I want to thank Reid Tracy, Nicolette Salamanca Young, and the entire Hay House family for believing in me and giving me the chance to write this book and share the Five Elements with parents and kids around the world!

ABOUT THE AUTHOR

Robin Ray Green, L.Ac., MTCM, is a California and national board-licensed acupuncturist and herbalist with a master's degree in Traditional Chinese Medicine from the prestigious Five Branches University in Santa Cruz, CA. She is a leading expert in the field of pediatric acupuncture with more than a decade of clinical experience helping children with asthma, allergies, and eczema heal using Chinese medicine.

Robin runs the popular kids' health blog, www.kidslove acupuncture.com, which has more than 1 million visitors annually. Her writing has been published in *Acupuncture Today, The California Journal of Oriental Medicine*, and other popular health blogs. A sought-after teacher, Robin founded the Center for Acupuncture Pediatrics, a premier training resource for pediatric acupuncture that supports acupuncturists worldwide.

Robin began her journey when her infant son came down with a severe, chronic case of eczema and Western medical treatments were unable to help him. In the process of healing her son, she realized her true calling was to help children and their parents integrate Chinese and Western medicine to facilitate healing. She believes that by using the ancient wisdom of Chinese medicine, we can heal many modern-day illnesses by strengthening the body with massage, diet, and lifestyle changes. She clears up the confusion about these natural treatments and helps parents create a custom healing program for their child—a program that supports many current medical treatments while safely and effectively using the tools of Chinese medicine to help the body heal itself.

When she's not working in her clinic, teaching, or writing, Robin enjoys bike riding with her family, playing at the beach, and walking her dog, Ginger. For more information about Robin and her work, please visit: www.robinraygreen.com.

Notes

Notes

We hope you enjoyed this Hay House book. If you'd like to receive our online catalog featuring additional information on Hay House books and products, or if you'd like to find out more about the Hay Foundation, please contact:

Hay House, Inc., P.O. Box 5100, Carlsbad, CA 92018-5100
(760) 431-7695 or (800) 654-5126
(760) 431-6948 (fax) or (800) 650-5115 (fax)
www.hayhouse.com® • www.hayfoundation.org

———

Published in Australia by: Hay House Australia Pty. Ltd.,
18/36 Ralph St., Alexandria NSW 2015
Phone: 612-9669-4299 • *Fax:* 612-9669-4144
www.hayhouse.com.au

Published in the United Kingdom by: Hay House UK, Ltd.,
The Sixth Floor, Watson House, 54 Baker Street, London W1U 7BU
Phone: +44 (0)20 3927 7290 • *Fax:* +44 (0)20 3927 7291
www.hayhouse.co.uk

Published in India by: Hay House Publishers India,
Muskaan Complex, Plot No. 3, B-2, Vasant Kunj, New Delhi 110 070
Phone: 91-11-4176-1620 • *Fax:* 91-11-4176-1630
www.hayhouse.co.in

———

Access New Knowledge.
Anytime. Anywhere.

Learn and evolve at your own pace
with the world's leading experts.

www.hayhouseU.com

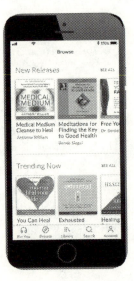

Printed in the United States
by Baker & Taylor Publisher Services